"Luna Grey has ___ ing look at the 21st-century BDSM scene from the straight-girl perspective, and her hard-won wisdom can help keep us all saner and safer." – Jay Wiseman, author, *SM 101: A Realistic Introduction, Tricks... To Please a Man*

"With wit, charm, and tons of good information, Luna Grey guides the newcomer through the twisted forest of introduction, negotiation and everything else you might need to know to play safe and explore your own wildness." – Dossie Easton, author, *The New Bottoming Book, The Ethical Slut*

"It's tough enough to face going to a beach with a new date for the first time. It's even tougher if you're a kinky girl and you have to explain the whip marks peeking out of your bikini from the previous night's butt-lashing. *The Kinky Girl's Guide to Dating* is a smart, irreverent, hilarious and playful manual that covers all the dilemmas those other dating books never get around to. No kinky girl should leave her dungeon without it." – Josey Vogels, sex and relationship columnist, *www.mymessybedroom.com*

the *kinky girl's*
guide to dating

the kinky girl's
guide to dating

by luna grey

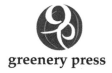

greenery press

Illustrations by Kimberly Schwede

Author photo by Sven Wiederholt

Published in the United States by Greenery Press, 3403 Piedmont Ave. #301, Oakland, CA 94611, *www.greenerypress.com*.

ISBN 1-890159-60-3.

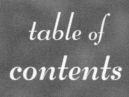

table of contents

Many thanks to all of my friends who listened to me process my mistakes when I made them the first time and then listened to me again when I prattled on endlessly during the writing of this book without shoving a gag down my throat. You know who you are. Thanks to all the people who lent me their experiences and insight. Thanks to Janet and Greenery Press for hearing my idea and then guiding me through making it into a reality. She was patient and compassionate when I was unproductive and equally patient when I was flooding her inbox. Thank you to "Suki" for writing her stories so beautifully and eloquently. Thank you to all the perverts who have shared my journeys, both good and bad, without whom I would have had nothing to write about.

To my parents, who taught me always to question the world around me, and to everyone who has the courage to walk their own path.

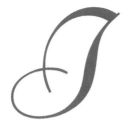 can't make this stuff up. The stories in this book are all based on truth, on stuff that happened to me or my friends or people I've talked to. They all have either my experiences or those of my friends at their cores. Extreme liberties have been taken with details and names have been changed to protect both the innocent and the not-so-innocent. The wackiest stories tend to be the closest to the truth. As I said, I can't make this stuff up.

BDSM is pansexual. Everyone does it. The stories in this book are primarily

foreword

hetero-oriented because that is my experience. Sadly, there isn't that much mixing between the leathermen, the hetero/bi scene, and the dykes, at least in San Francisco. Maybe people will be inspired and write *The Kinky Man's Guide to Dating* and *The Kinky Dyke's Guide to Dating,* etc. I hope so. I'd do it myself but unless my life takes some very unexpected twists, I'm not qualified!

Most, but not all, of this stuff happened in the SF Bay area. Some stuff about the scene, typical party rules, some etiquette details, vary regionally. YMMV (Your Mileage May Vary).

As you'll see, there are three basic types of material in here. You'll hear most from one lady, "Maddie." No, she's not me, although we have an awful lot in common. She's part me, part my best buddies, and part every other fumbling struggling wannabe submissive woman who's ever tried to hide a paddle mark with pancake makeup before a gynecologist appointment.

You'll also hear a few hair-raising tales from my dear friend "Suki," a novice dominant. I thought being a submissive was tough until Suki started sharing her tales of woe. Now I think pro-dommes don't get paid nearly enough.

And finally, you'll hear me talking in my own voice – just me, Luna. If you get lost, look up at the top of the page to find out whether you're reading about Maddie or Suki or whether it's just me giving my opinions again.

I'm not a therapist, a counselor, a doctor, or any other sort of qualified professional. I'm just a girl who has been around this stuff for a while. I've thought about it, discussed it, read about it, and done it *a lot*. While this book may be a jumping-off point, I would highly suggest also reading some other BDSM how-to books that go into safety rules and practices much more deeply than I do. I have merely scratched the surface to show you that such rules and standards exist.

Enjoy, play safe, and come hard and often!
Luna Grey

Maddie's path to discovery was a gradual process suddenly hastened by the Internet in the early 1990s. The fact that there were other people out there who had these fantasies, that it was not just fodder for erotica, but actually a reality... well, that was a revelation that just about blew off the top of her skull. The options seemed endless and they rolled out in front of her like a glorious red carpet of sexual possibility. She had no idea how many wrinkles were in that carpet for her to rather ingloriously stumble over.

*she **remembers** the teacher finding her tied up to the swing set...*

She'd been kinky for pretty much as long as she could remember. She remembered – was it in kindergarten? – the teacher finding her tied up to the swing set at the end of recess. She didn't just play "doctor" as a young child, she played mad scientist.

Her version was pretty dark, involving elaborate punishment scenes in a neighbor's basement. Not surprisingly, she was usually the one who got punished. She has a half-formed memory of having a bucket of

1

coal poured over her crotch while she moaned and writhed in semi-protest. She can still remember the absolute feeling of erotic surrender, the feeling of loss of control. That memory has a sexual charge for her even now, sparking over the years. These dirty little games continued until the inevitable discovery by a parent at which point they abruptly ceased. She doesn't remember seeing those kids much after that.

The games went on in the schoolyard… elaborate scenarios involving cowboys and wild horses. Maddie, dragged into captivity, happily kicking and screaming. Again, inevitably, interrupted by pesky adults when her struggles became too vigorous, the screams too loud and realistic-sounding.

During the teenage years, her sexual awakening seemed to always involve some sort of power exchange dynamic. She chose older boys… the dangerous ones… who would use her. And she submitted to this, sometimes with great drama but some weird little part of her loved it… loved feeling used and possessed even as she bemoaned it. The pain of losing her virginity was one of the hottest moments of her life. Unhealthy? Hell, yeah. Self-destructive? Absolutely. It's sort of like a gay kid trying and trying to get aroused with the op-

KINKY GIRL TIP

watch these spaces for kinky girl tips throughout the book!

KINKY GIRL TIP

posite gender while secretly harboring very different fantasies and not understanding their own behaviors until much later. She tried the nice guys, but oh... the bad ones always got her in the end.

In college she got clever and started using props. Now, none of it was kinky, mind you... just... well... *interesting*. She just thought she was being progressive. Vibrators, blindfolds, hot wax, ice cubes, heating creams. The first time someone used handcuffs on her, she was so aroused she almost swallowed her own tongue. She went out to the local hardware store the next day and bought her own set because that was definitely something she needed to have around. They were a cheap pair that cut the wrists and later fell into pieces but at the time, they were the be-all and end-all of kinkiness to her. The first time she pulled the handcuffs out, the guy thought they were for him and she looked at him, completely baffled as to how to give him the right idea. She didn't have the wherewithal to actually ask for what she wanted. Negotiating certainly wasn't part of the vocabulary and asking for it seemed too much like admitting something she wasn't ready to admit.

Then she made the radical mistake of moving to the Deep South for graduate school. Now, the South has many things going for it. Easy winters, good deep-

3

fried food, beautiful beaches… but good ribs or not, it is quite definitely *not* the place to discover that you're in any way aberrant sexually. So, of course, that's where Maddie figured it out.

It felt like Christmas, she just didn't have anyone to play with her new toys with her. She was so earnest about it all and was fortunate enough to have some rather tolerant, if somewhat uncomprehending, gay male friends who remembered their own "coming-out" process. She was *proud.* She bought all of the pride jewelry, put the leather pride sticker on her car, got some outfits comprised mainly of leather and chains and wore them out dancing in the gay clubs.

She did everything a novice pervert can do when isolated in the Deep South. She read every book on the subject that she could order on-line. She met people over the Internet. She went home on vacations and played with people in New York. Then she moved to Mecca, that light at the end of the tunnel: San Francisco.

I remember learning about drugs when I was a kid. The party line was that if you try marijuana, even *once*, you will end up a heroin addict on the streets, giving five-dollar blowjobs to support the monkey on your back. The road to ruin was inevitable once you take that first baby step. You will have no choice in the matter.

Maybe wanting to tempt fate, I did try smoking pot, I even inhaled. It was fine. That road to ruin didn't appear

at my feet. I just got high. I did it again. My life continued. I went to school, got into college, eventually got
bored with smoking pot and didn't do it any more. I chose
when and where and how much. I satisfied my cu-
riosity and then I moved on.

People getting into BDSM (a weird acronym:
bondage/discipline, dominance/submission,
sadism/masochism – who thought *that* one
up?) sometimes have the same fears, that
they will lose all choice

KINKY GIRL TIP

If you can, spend a couple of
minutes before you play just
breathing quietly, centering
yourself and letting the
worries of the day slip away.
It may not seem sexy, but it
pays off later by making you
more relaxed and responsive.

KINKY GIRL TIP

in the matter, that once you take the first step off the
vanilla path, you're doomed. You will end up covered
in tattoos and piercings, living your life clad only in
leather (or latex, or PVC, depending on your bent). You
will descend into this underground world of deviant
sexuality, live your life in the shadows of twisted eroti-
cism, never be able to cope with regular society again,
rejected by friends and family. You get the picture.

The road is yours to create. There are no inevitable
outcomes. You can choose what you want to experiment
with and how far you want to go. You may find that your
comfort levels expand, that you want to try more and
more extreme activities. You may discover that this isn't
really for you. You may experiment for a while and then

quit. You may find the niche of BDSM sexuality where you feel comfortable and settle in quite happily.

The world of sexuality is enormous and varied. If you can step outside the narrow boundaries proscribed by society, you may find pleasures you had only imagined. You have to remember that you are in control of where you want to go. Stay safe, stay sane, make sure that you pay attention to your own comfort levels. Use common sense.

You can live a perfectly normal life day-to-day and experiment with being kinky in your private time. A scarlet "P" for pervert will not appear on your forehead. You are not required to wear fetishwear to work and pierce every flap of skin on your body. You are in control of who you choose to share this part of your life with.

Can you be a feminist and a submissive? Absolutely. On the surface it may seem like a contradiction in terms: how can a strong independent woman hand over control to someone else? The important thing is to realize that you are not really handing over the ultimate control unless you are in an abusive situation. The submissive always has the final word in what happens to her. You are actually owning your sexuality. You are leaving the blueprint given to you by others. You are making choices and negotiating for what you want. Nothing is more strong and independent than that.

Being in control of your own sexuality, as opposed to letting society dictate what it *should* be, can be a very empowering experience. Create the path that you want to go down for yourself.

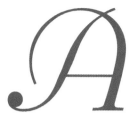

All right, so you've figured out that you're kinky. Now you need to find people who share your tastes, people to either slap you around or who you can slap around. They are out there, you are not alone. Unfortunately, kinky folks don't wear labels. Frequently the biggest pervert can look like the most conservative guy or girl next door. So what avenues do you take?

The Internet has revolutionized how people find each other. Looking online can be your first step. Many communities have BDSM organizations, particularly urban areas. The Society of Janus

1: *how to search for partners*

in San Francisco, The Eulenspiegel Society in New York. Please see the Resource Guide at the back of this book for ways to find other regional groups. Many times, these societies offer classes, have parties, sponsor conventions, have email lists for members, etc. That can be one route for finding your community.

Munches, another great way of meeting people, are informal gatherings in a neutral space like a restaurant. People get together to chat and socialize in a low-key environment. It's a great way for newcomers to meet people and get information on the local scene.

You can also look for your local fetish clubs or events. Sometimes newcomers find this a little bit intimidating and it can be difficult to just meet people and chat at these events. They may be better left until you have met some people in the scene – then you can go with a girlfriend, or with a male friend that you haven't "clicked" with romantically, so you have someone to hang out with and it feels a little less scary.

On-line dating is another way to go. There are personals websites dedicated to the BDSM community, such as *alt.com* and *bondage.com.* As with all online dating sites, one needs to take precautions when meeting strangers off the Internet – more about this later. Kinky people can also be found on some of the vanilla sites, but one has to be more attuned to some more subtle clues in the wording of the ads. If you are posting an ad yourself, it helps to be very specific about what you are looking for and also be very honest about what your own level of experience is.

There are a lot of BDSM chatrooms out there. Remember, anyone can call themselves Master Dom of the Universe online. You may well be talking to a 14-year-old boy who found his parents' erotica collection. While it might be a fun way to kill a couple of hours or play out a fantasy in a safe arena, it often has very little connection to reality. People can get pretty involved with it, Tops always referring to themselves in capital letters, bottoms in lower case, cyber "collarings," online "scening," etc. It's sort of like an interactive kinky video game of sorts, "Everquest" for perverts or wannabe-perverts. In my opinion, this is not a great way to meet people. Many folks who spend a lot of time in BDSM chatrooms aren't spending a lot of time doing this in real life, if any at all. A dead giveaway is anyone who opens a conversation with a variant of "Kneel before me now, worthless slut." "You ain't the boss of me," "Eat my shorts," or "You first" are some handy responses.

While you can get to know somebody to an extent by email, chatting online and on the phone, you just never *know* until you meet them. I once chatted with someone for a couple of months; we got along very well, seemed to click. We finally arranged to meet and it was just "wrong." He had this sort of deranged look in his eyes and he just smelled "off." Not bad, mind you, but I'll blame it on pheromones. I told him that I thought the chemistry was wrong and he proceeded to get pretty nasty. That deranged look in his eyes got even more deranged and I got the hell out of there. Some friends of mine have developed perfectly healthy relationships online before they actually met but I'm a big fan of setting up a safe face-to-face meeting pretty quickly. I'm a busy girl and I find it saves time. To this end, I don't try to date long-distance. I don't want to get all involved with someone who lives across the country only to waste money on a plane ticket and decide that he smells wrong too. That's a decision you have to make for yourself.

When finding people, one thing to consider is whether or not they are part of the local BDSM community. If they are out and about to at least some extent, you can find out what their reputation in the scene is and you might even get to see how they play at a party. As in any community, the members become accountable for their actions, a known element. Once you start networking in the BDSM community, you will be surprised at how easy it is to build a social group.

There are also BDSM conventions like Black Rose and Fire in the Mountains. Think lots of perverts, toys, clothes, classes, lectures, demos, and parties. Rock on.

Another nice thing about meeting people who are in the BDSM community is that you can get references on them. It is a fairly common practice to ask someone if there is anyone who will give them a reference. What we're playing with can be dangerous and this is a way of trying to stay safe. They can speak with their other play partners, check if it is all right with them and then put you in touch with them. There are issues of confidentiality in the scene, people like to control how much they are "out." Standard etiquette is that you don't talk about playing with someone to a third party without that person's permission.

You also need to be careful that your source is reliable. I once got a good reference on someone and had a disastrous experience with them. I hadn't known the woman who had given me the reference very well and I later figured out she wasn't all there. Likewise, if you chat with someone's ex, and they had a bad breakup, you may get a very biased opinion. (Be especially careful of *unsolicited* references – if someone makes a point about warning you about X before you've even asked, they may have an ax to grind.) Use your good judgment, ask more than one person, and try to do your homework wisely.

*R*yan is a nice guy. Maddie had met him around the scene years ago and then hadn't seen him for a little while. He reappeared at a munch. He is more attractive than she remembered and she gives him her phone number. They go out for dinner and it is well... *nice.* No fireworks... no sparks flying back and forth... but she doesn't want to be too hasty dismissing him. It has been a while since she has met anyone who captures her interest even a little. The same faces seem to be showing up at the various events again and again. San Francisco,

she thought she'd give him the benefit of the doubt...

supposedly one of the hubs of BDSM activity, is starting to feel like a small pond.

He walks her to her door and then she invites him in. He reaches out and strokes the nape of her neck and suddenly she feels the beginning of something. Some sparks? Maybe there is some chemistry after all or maybe it's just some weird Pavlovian response to his touch on her neck, an automatic response to an erogenous zone. They end up on her

11

couch and that's when things start to go wrong. The kiss, for starters: his lips are like two slugs wrestling limply. She wants to be kissed so that she forgets all reason. "Be patient," she thinks, "maybe it will get better as he relaxes." It doesn't.

He starts to growl. Growling can be effective, done properly. A low bass rumble... the purr of a large cat about to devour a meal. His growling is more like a peeved puppy and she is appalled. Laughter rises almost involuntarily and threatens to spill out but is stifled by another one of his wet kisses. 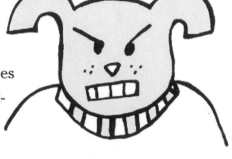 When she emerges, she looks up at him in dismay.

He misinterprets what he sees in her eyes. "You want to submit," he says in a voice much deeper than his normal speaking tone, the basso profundo of masterful conviction, "but you're afraid."

He got part of it right: she is afraid. She is afraid there is no graceful way to get him off her couch and out of the apartment. How to do it without wounding his fragile dominant ego. How to not reveal how ridiculous she finds the entire situation. He is just so *nice*. Growling and ridiculous, but sort of sweet. She wishes the couch would just swallow her whole so she can disappear. Better yet, she wishes the couch would swallow *him*.

She chooses the easy way out. She cringes inwardly at her cowardice but she's just too tired to deal with brutal honesty.

"Ummm... I'm afraid this is going too fast... it's too powerful."

He backs off immediately if somewhat reluctantly.

"I just need... I need to be able to think and I can't do that right now... with all this...." She trails off, hoping he will think she means she is befuddled by his dominance and power.

It works. He is a perfect gentleman and leaves... saying it is "inevitable" that they will see each other again.

When he calls the next day, she recognizes his number on her caller ID and almost doesn't answer the phone. Then she rebukes herself and takes the call. "Hello?"

"Hey," he says, "How are you?"

"I'm fine... busy...." And a coward, she adds to herself.

"Oh. Well, it's nothing important. I just wanted to tell you what a great time I had last night."

"It was nice," she says, wincing and waiting for the inevitable.

"So I was wondering, when can I see you again?"

She curses herself for not dealing with this the previous night. "Look, I just... I'm looking for a long-term relationship, and I really like you, but I just don't

13

see the potential for that with us." She hears herself babbling and trails off.

There's a brief silence on the other end of the phone. Then he says, "Well, I'm kind of surprised. I thought we had chemistry." Like a lab experiment gone horribly wrong, she thinks.

"I know," she stammers. "I'm sorry."

"I'm sorry too," he answers slowly. "I guess I'll see you around."

There will be no more growling.

How wide do you cast your net when you're looking for play partners? If you see someone and your pelvis doesn't explode with an immediate flare of panty-drenching lust, does it still have a chance of working out? Is your Prince Charming exactly 6'1" and 180 lbs. with shoulder-length black hair, a sculpted bod, and green eyes, and you won't settle for anything less?

Tough question. Sometimes the most erotic connections can spring up in the most unexpected places. I met one guy who was about fifty years old, had a long gray beard, and weighed about

> **KINKY GIRL TIP**
>
> A little tasteful perfume can be lovely but if your top's eyes are watering and he's sneezing it will screw up his aim. Tone it down.
>
> **KINKY GIRL TIP**

350 pounds. Not exactly what I would have considered my physical ideal. But I got to know him and ended up playing with him for quite a while. He was a wonderful kind man, an astoundingly skilled and clever top, a very sexy guy, and a major part of one of the most erotic chapters in my life. He moved and then I moved and I haven't seen him for years, but I am still grateful to him. I was very very lucky to have run into him when I was new to the scene.

I guess what I'm trying to say is that if you hold out for a very specific physical ideal, you might miss out on some fabulous experiences.

Now if you're just plain not attracted to someone, don't push it in the hopes that maybe something will develop. Either it will or it won't. There will be people out there in the scene that you may not ever want to play with but they will be great friends, or mentors, or people that you can go to play parties with because you just don't feel like walking in the door alone. As in any area of life, there will also be people you just flat-out don't like.

Don't get desperate and start playing with people you have no connection to whatsoever because chances are they'll start growling and you'll be left cold and trying to figure how to get them out the door. Maybe this guy would have been a great friend for Maddie but she blew it by trying to play with him when the connection wasn't there. Hard to develop a friendship after that.

Keep an open mind about what is sexy to you. We've been bombarded with media images about who

15

is supposed to appear sexy to us (this is something I can rant on about at length but I'll restrain myself... heh... I said "restrain myself"). You may find you're wet for a certain look in someone's eyes rather than six-pack abs.

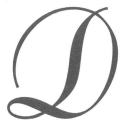ear Maddie,

Well, I've had my first playdate – at least I suppose you could call it that. I guess next week I'll figure out whether to laugh or cry about it. For now, I'll just say that this was the evening that they wrote the expression "careful what you wish for" about.

So, as you know, I met the guy for coffee last week, and I spent the past week trying to work up a bit more attraction for him, but it just wasn't there, at least not much. He was just Joe Average – average height, a bit chubby, not dressed all that well, needed a haircut. Not bad, not great, just, well, you know.

> "he lay there *wheezing* like an asthmatic *trampoline*..."

But how many guys are going to be interested in letting a woman take them over her knees and spank them? I mean, really? I've been dreaming about this for *such* a long time... so I spent the week fantasizing about it, and the hell with whether I was all that turned on by *him* or not, I was just plain *turned on*.

And then, just a couple of days before the big date, my package showed up from that website you and I looked at, and lord only knows what the postman thought – how many packages does he deliver that are four inches across and thirty inches long, do you suppose? But there it was, my very own cane, just like in all the Victorian porn. Honestly, Maddie, it didn't look like all that much – just a thin, bendy stick with varnish on it, with leather wrapped around it at one end. How much would a thing like that hurt? So I figured I'd better find out. I took hold of the handle and gave myself a good whack on the thigh over my jeans – and let out a squawk that should have shattered all the wine glasses on my kitchen shelves, and threw the nasty thing all the way across the dining room. Oh my *god* it hurt! And even through my jeans it left a big dark-red welt all the way across my thigh.

It's still lying in the corner of my dining room. I'm sort of afraid to touch it again.

So, needless to say, the cane didn't come along on my big playdate. But everything else did – a nice bag with my ping-pong paddle, my hairbrush, some ropes, a blindfold, that little buttplug and the lube I bought at the sex shop, everything I thought I might need.

And I dressed in my highest heels (what moron decided that high heels were supposed to make a woman look powerful? – they make me feel like a ten-month-old trying to learn to walk), and black stockings and a short skirt, and all that stuff. And dark lipstick, and my hair up. And in the mirror, I looked just like the dominant women in the magazines, and I thought this was all going to be great, just like in my fantasies. And I was wet even before I left the house.

And when I got there, he didn't look all that bad. He was wearing pretty good clothes, a dark blue button-down shirt and nice jeans, and he'd had a haircut. And, frankly, I was so turned on by then that Frankenstein's Monster could have shown up and I'd have told him to drop trou.

So we got checked in – and thanks again for being my safecall – and there we were, in this motel room. And I hadn't really thought this part through. My imagination had kind of skipped to the part where he was already pants-down and over my knees; I had no real idea how he was going to get there. We just sort of stared at each other for a while. I don't suppose it was really more than sixty seconds or so, but, Maddie, it seemed like a month and a half.

Finally, I stammered out, "So, naughty boy. I think it's time you took your pants down." (Something like that, any-way. I think I probably sounded about as authoritative as a fourth-grader on the first day of school.)

He looked at me oddly for a moment, but then kind of shrugged and took off his jeans and underpants and stood there with his dick hanging there. I took his arm, backed into a chair and pulled him across my lap – well, at least *that* part felt more or less like the fantasies, al-though I'd never realized how large a grown man is and how hard it is to fit a whole one onto your lap; they tend to sort of ooze off the edges of your knees. But anyway, I started smacking away at his chubby butt with my hand, and then when my hand got sore (another part that hadn't really happened in the fantasy), with the ping pong paddle.

And he just sort of lay there. He twitched a little bit at some of the harder smacks, but it was pretty obvious that

19

this wasn't doing a thing for him. I began to feel a little bit like one of those women on the Discovery Channel who pounds laundry on flat rocks. If I'd had an erection, it would have gone totally limp by now. I gently shoved him off my lap and he stood up.

"Can we try something else now?" he asked.

"Um, sure," I said. (Is this some new definition of "dominance" I haven't heard about yet?)

He yanked off his shirt so he was now totally naked, and flopped face up on the floor. "Walk on me," he demanded.

"Uh – what?" I stammered.

"Come on, *walk* on me," he repeated, sounding a little pissed off this time.

> **KINKY GIRL TIP**
>
> Ladies, if you're topping, figure out what you want to be called and tell your bottom. Ma'am? Goddess? Your Highness? Milady? Mistress? Master? Sir? Daddy? The poor thing can get very confused otherwise.
>
> **KINKY GIRL TIP**

"Oh, OK, sure, I guess. Lemme take my shoes off," I said.

"Geeze, I thought you said you were dominant. Leave the shoes *on*," he said, now clearly annoyed.

Eeek. I'm not a lightweight, and those heels are *high* and not exactly chunky. Just in case, I grabbed a nearby table with one hand and gingerly stepped on board.

It was sort of like pressing a button on a machine. The minute he felt the sole of my shoe sink into his chest, his head dropped back, his face turned pink, his eyes closed ecstatically, his dick rose like the striped pole at a railroad crossing, and he started to breathe hard. Of course, that didn't make it any easier keeping my balance.

Well, getting walked on by 160 lbs. of very confused novice domme was clearly It for him. I teetered from his collarbone down to his dick – and, yes, dear, he even had me step on his dick, although I wouldn't do it as hard as he wanted me to – and back again. And for good measure, I planted my size-eight right on his open mouth while he wheezed like an asthmatic trampoline.

Where were all those "I only want to please you, Mistress" subs I've been reading about? This guy didn't give a shit whether he was pleasing me or not as long as he got to go home with a bunch of Suki-prints all over his front.

And for good measure, as he was getting dressed, he hinted shyly that his *last* girlfriend used to step on bugs for him. Oh ick ick ick *ick*. Honest, all I wanted to do was wallop someone's ass. Is that so much to ask?

There is clearly much more to this sexual dominance business than meets the eye. I sure hope it's easier from your end than it seems to be from mine.

Much love and much confusion,

Suki

People are into things you can't even imagine. Before playing with them, during the negotiation process, it is a good idea to try to figure out what their buttons are. This isn't always easy and if they're new, they may not even know themselves. You may not be totally clear on what exactly it is that you want. But your buttons may not be theirs.

21

There are a million different ways to top someone. Just because you're a top and they're a bottom does not mean that the two of you will have the hottest interactions since the destruction of Pompeii. Poor Suki was left with her mouth hanging open. Walking on her partner left her literally off-balance and dry as the Sahara.

The discovery process between two people can be fun and exciting. Finding someone's turn-ons, *especially* if they didn't know about them, can be the hottest thing imaginable. Many people like playing with "newbies" because they enjoy opening up new worlds for them and seeing their eyes light up at the new sensations, new feelings they had never even imagined. But you have to have a sense of humor about the whole thing. Being comfortable with the other person helps so that you can laugh about it together when something doesn't click and talk openly and honestly to figure out what will.

Try asking about their fantasies. You can even have them write you a story. This guy would probably have written about being used as a sidewalk and Suki would either have worn more sensible shoes or decided that she really just wasn't that interested. She wanted to smack someone's bottom. Whether she knew it or not, there are plenty of bottoms out there to smack. Hell, there are entire groups of people out there who are purely into spanking. If Suki had happened upon one of those folks, she might have had a great scene.

The world of BDSM is vast and sometimes that gets forgotten. Just because you're both kinky does not mean that you have anything in common sexually *at all* beyond the fact that what you're into falls outside the narrow norms of our society. It takes a little work and communication to figure out if you're compatible play partners or not.

I was once at a discussion group and someone asked a new submissive woman what she was into. "Oh", she said with a glazed look in her wide eyes, "I'm into *everything*. I want to try it *all*." The older players grinned and began to offer suggestions. Scat play? Branding? Being hung upside down and covered with honey and ants? Enemas? The woman looked very startled and started to stammer. It was gently pointed out to her that maybe she needed to do some reading and start out slow. Possibly she would end up actually being into all those things but she hadn't even realized they were options. It turned out that her idea of BDSM had encompassed a rather narrow range of activities. She needed to learn to set some limits during negotiations or else she would find things being done to her that she certainly hadn't fantasized about.

> **KINKY GIRL TIP**
>
> Practice walking in those new stilettos at home before you debut them in public. Remember, weight on the ball of your foot.
>
> **KINKY GIRL TIP**

The choice not to take the cane was a very wise one on Suki's part. She had wanted it, had fantasized about it, but when it arrived, she realized that it was something she wasn't qualified to use yet. That was a remarkably clear-minded decision for someone so new. While her scene was uncomfortable and embarrassing, no one got injured. The best single-tail artist I have ever met practiced for a year on balloons and pillows before he ever used his whip on human flesh. It is important to remember that any idiot can go buy a very dangerous toy, no waiting period, no knowledge or skill required. Even toys that don't look dangerous can do some serious damage. Play with people who know what they're doing. If you're topping, know when you're not qualified to use your shiny new toy on an actual human being. Practice, go to classes, read books, watch people who *do* know what they're doing. Most of all, be patient. When you're ready to use it, chances are there will be someone around who would be happy to have it used on them.

Suki made another wise choice when she used Maddie as her safecall. Safecalls are very important. So important that I might just put this in capital letters: SAFECALLS ARE VERY IMPORTANT. Got it? Now, you might be asking, what the hell is a "safecall" and why is she shouting about it? A safecall is kind of a safety net. Find someone reliable and tell them where you will be and who you will be with and all the information you have on that person – their legal name, address, phone number, email address, the whole thing. Next, come up with a time, or a series or times, that you will check in with them. For the more paranoid, you might even set up an innocuous code word that means "I'm

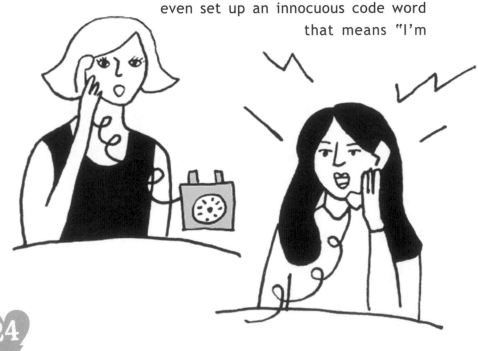

in trouble" and another one that means "I'm fine." Tell your safecall person what you want them to do if you don't check in. Try calling you on your cell phone and at home. Call your spouse? Call your parents? Tell them at what point in the proceedings you want them to call the police. Basically, what you are doing is setting up a chain of events that will go into motion if you don't check in. You should set up a safecall for not just the first coffee date, but the first few dates. Definitely for the first time you will be in a private space with this person.

Then, the most important step: *Tell your date that you've done all that.* Tell him in advance that you're going to, if you want to be careful about confidentiality. How this plays out is like this: "Oh, by the way. Before I go out with someone for the first time, I always give my best friend a piece of paper with the guy's name and address on it, and let her know when I'm expected back. I hope that's not a problem for you. She's completely trustworthy, of course." This can be a little bit awkward, but in a way it's your first big litmus test: if the guy throws a hissy fit over it, you should be hearing big alarm bells over whether or not this guy is safe enough for you to be seeing at all. If he's a complete novice, he may never have heard of such a thing and be understandably a little weirded out by the whole idea, but once you explain that you're just looking out for your own safety he should understand. Offer your own information in exchange, of course. I've even heard of a few tops who instruct their new submissives to set up safecalls as part of their instructions about what to do, wear, etc., on their first dates (bravo!!).

I once was someone's safecall. The system kind of collapsed because we both flaked. She didn't call but I had completely forgotten as well. Fortunately she was just having a lot of orgasms. So, pick someone more reliable than I am and remember to make your safecall or the cops may well come knocking.

Remember, safecalls are not just for submissives (and not just for women – don't be surprised if it turns out that your date has set one up too!). Dommes need them too. Yes, I know, you're the one in control, what could possibly happen to you? But remember, you have to untie them eventually and it's tough to run fast in stilettos.

Of course, if you find yourself in a really dangerous position, trust your instinct and call 911. Don't worry about explaining an embarrassing situation to the police. Cops have seen everything and your safety is worth a little embarrassment.

addie met Mitchell at a "kinky speed dating" event. She had five minutes with each of fifteen different guys. When the guy was interesting and attractive, five minutes didn't seem like a long time as the conversation flowed through it too quickly. When the man across from her was about as entertaining as a dead sea slug and she caught herself counting his nose hairs, the five minutes stretched out into a small eternity.

With Mitchell she had wanted the conversation to continue. He

> *"they **must** paint their fingernails and **toenails** purple..."*

had a laugh that seemed to emanate out of the very core of him. She checked "yes" next to his number on the contact sheet they handed out at the event. A day later, she was pleased to receive an email from the dating service with his contact information.

He wrote her a couple of very polite and articulate emails, asking more about her, quietly flirtatious without being offensive. She wrote back and even allowed herself to get a little bit excited. She was pleased whenever she found a note from him in her inbox. It had been a while since she had met some-one she was interested in. She was usually cautious with her enthusiasm: years in the scene had left her slightly jaded and used to disappointment. Maybe she was just too critical. (A book she'd read recently had made her wonder if she was contributing to her own dismal relationship history: *"A fear of commit-ment on your part drives you to choose inappropriate partners."* She disliked self-help books in general, and this one in particular rang a little too true. She hid it under a pile of sweaters and didn't finish it.)

Finally Mitchell calls to set up an appointment to meet for coffee. Maddie mentally hushes the voices in her head as she gets dressed and does her makeup, *"What's wrong with this one? You know there'll be something."* She dresses carefully, a new skirt, heels because, heavens be praised, he is tall enough that she can wear them and still look up at him. She straightens her hair with an iron so that it swings in a curtain around her face.

He stands as she enters the busy coffeeshop, kisses her cheek and holds her chair for her. So far, so good. He is a gentleman – but she felt the touch of his eyes as they stroked up and down her body. Gloria Steinem be damned, she likes that.

He starts the conversation with inconsequential trivia. They speak about the neighborhood, various coffeeshops they both like. He laughs that wonderful laugh and leans in to touch her arm. His hands are warm. When she looks away, she feels him studying her.

The conversation gradually turns to BDSM. He asks how long she has been involved with it. She cringes inwardly, almost lies, then tells the truth and watches carefully for his reaction. She has been involved in the kinky world for about eight years. Some tops don't like that: it's like saying you have a greater level of sexual experience than they do. One top had told her he was intimidated and would prefer someone who was newer, and made her feel like fruit that had been on the tree too long and was starting to turn soft and black at the middle. Mitchell sails right through this test – he has been in the scene for about twenty years and has no problem with experienced submissives.

KINKY GIRL TIP

Yeah, everyone wants to be a movie star but before you let someone take X-rated pictures or video, remember that the Internet exists. Two words: Paris Hilton. Use your best judgment.

KINKY GIRL TIP

Was it possible? Was this one actually the unicorn she had been seeking?

Then he says he has five things he likes new submissives to "do for him."

Oh no. Little bells start to ring faintly in her head and the little voices hiss in triumphant delight. She gamely ignores them and asks what those five things are.

At this point, he veers rather abruptly off the path of possibility and lands ungracefully on the heap of no hope.

1. They must paint their fingernails and toenails purple.

2. They must shave their pussies and keep them bare.

3. They must never wear underpants.

4. They must pierce their nipples.

5. They must never say "no" to any reasonable request.

The voices in Maddie's head are shrieking a delighted chorus of *"I told you so!"* while she absorbs his list. Her pussy is already shaved and she frequently goes without panties because she likes the feeling of secret naughtiness – no big deal, really. But purple nailpolish makes her look like a drowning victim who had been in the water for a while.

Her brain stumbles over the fourth item as if it were sticking on a scratched CD. She struggles to keep a polite expression on her face. Pierce her nipples? A major body modification is a prerequisite? How many women had gone to piercing parlors for this guy? She'd had her nipples pierced before and they had been a major inconvenience for three years before she finally removed them. She still remembers blood dripping down her chest like tears after someone played with them a little too roughly. Does he care?

Number five on his list causes the train to derail completely. "They must never say 'no' to any reasonable request." After all, this is a man who has nipple piercing as a requirement for *everybody* he plays with. Presumably he thinks that *is* a reasonable request.

While the little voices dance their mad jig of howling victory, Maddie stands up. She smiles at him and says simply, "We're looking for very different things. Good luck in your search." She shakes his hand and walks away. She drives home with her unpierced nipples and deletes his emails. Disappointment trickles through her in a small blue stream.

I used to stammer and balk about saying no. I was raised in a New England family where tact was rather highly prized. I would sometimes not say no when I should have. I would string out second chances indefinitely with people I knew to be inappropriate. I wanted to please, not to disappoint or hurt feelings. I tried to do things gracefully. Unfortunately it was frequently at the cost of my personal integrity.

Once I slept with a man because I had gone home with him and his bed was the only clean spot in the house. The whole place was an utter disaster and smelled like old fish. The second I walked in, the only thing I could think about was getting out – but I couldn't figure out how. I had said yes when he crushed me up against the car and kissed me. I had said yes when he tangled his fingers in the hair at the nape of my neck and pulled. I had said yes when he had invited me back to his place to fool around. When I saw his house (and smelled it) I wanted to scream *no,* but I didn't want to hurt his feelings. I couldn't figure it out and the sheets were clean – so I slept with him and escaped as quickly as I could, not wanting to touch anything, and went home to wash the odor of rotting tidepools out of my hair.

Sometimes you have to hurt people's feelings, to disappoint, in order to maintain your boundaries and say no. It can be more difficult if your entire sexual identity is structured around pleasing the person that you're with, but it can still be done.

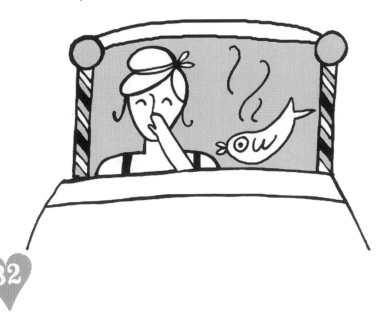

Be very tuned in to your own comfort levels. When you start feeling uncomfortable, pay attention to that right away. Don't tamp it down and wait to see if it gets better. Chances are, it won't. Take it out and examine it. Hold it up to the light and turn it over and see if you can find where it emanates from.

If you're on a date with someone you're unsure about, give yourself a "time out." Go to the bathroom and figure out what is going on. Then figure out how you can regain your comfort zone. Possibly ask for a point to be clarified if you think you may have misunderstood something he has said.

Submissive or not, you can always say no at any point in the proceedings. I always like to arrive separately and have my car with me on the first few dates so that I can leave alone. I still struggle with tact versus honesty. You do not need to go into elaborate explanations. My father, bless his heart, once told me that women frequently feel the need to explain when they say no, to apologize, quantify and clarify when a simple no should suffice.

I should have walked into that man's house, said "I'm afraid this isn't going to work out," and left. It might have been awkward but certainly no more awkward than having sex with him. Fucking someone or playing with them simply to be polite is, to put it mildly, going overboard.

Your "no" may not always be well-received by potential partners. Use that to shore up the bastion or your refusal. *The worse their reaction, the more assurance that you are doing the right thing.* Be polite but be firm and remember you do not have to explain. They may ask for an explanation and you can be as honest as you want to be. You can tell them that you can't stand being in those surroundings, that you think it is possibly indicative of their internal order, that you hate the smell of fish, that you don't want to be with someone who requires you to pierce your nipples. Or you can just say that you don't have the words to explain it, you just need to say no.

Struggling with discomfort just to avoid the awkwardness of the refusal will just get you deeper into the situation, wasting your time and his. While you are perfectly justified to say no whenever you want to, in my experience, it's easier to get it over with early on. Don't wait until the needles are about to go through.

Maddie meets Ilana and George at one of the first munches she goes to. They seem like such, well, normal people. People she might have gone to college with, or met in a café or the library. Ilana teaches second grade and she is short and curvy, with twinkling eyes under a mop of irrepressible brown hair. George is tall and lanky, a lawyer, and he watches his wife with an air of bemused affection as she bounces around the room. Maddie takes to them both immediately. She goes out to coffee with Ilana and talks about coming

"even the ones yelling in pain seem to be having such a good time!"

into the whole BDSM thing. Ilana laughs a lot and tells funny stories about her own discovery process. She met George through the local BDSM organization five years ago. Maddie wonders who's the top in the relationship until Ilana tells her. Ilana, this bubbly, opinionated woman, calls herself "submissive."

She leans close to Maddie, "He's vicious," she confides, "I *love* it." Maddie has a hard time picturing the bespectacled affable guy she met being "vicious."

35

One day Ilana calls her, "Hey, we're going to a play party on Friday night. Do you want to come along? I don't think we're going to play but there's a bunch of people that we want to see." Maddie hesitates for a moment, her stomach churning. Images rush through her brain of cold intimidating people, clad all in fetishwear in a dark cavelike dungeon. "Ummm... I don't know..." she hedges, "I've never been..."

Ilana is smiling, she can hear it in her voice, "I know, sweetie. This would be the perfect opportunity to get your toes wet. If you're uncomfortable, we'll leave and go get dinner somewhere. No harm, no foul. George'll be fine with it."

"OK," Maddie says before she can think about it too much, "I'd like that."

"Great! We'll pick you up at eight on Friday. Feel free to call in the meantime if you have any questions."

"Wait!" Maddie says, "What should I wear?!"

Ilana laughs, "Always the problem, isn't it? Wear what you're comfortable in. I'm going to shake the dust off of my corset because I never get to wear it but this isn't a high fetish party. There will be people there in fetishwear and people there in jeans."

Maddie's brain is already feverishly combing her closet. "OK, I'll see you Friday... and thanks!"

It's Friday night, 7:30, and the contents of Maddie's closet are strewn across her bedroom. She's focusing on clothes so she can ignore the relentless butterflies in her stomach. She's turned on by this whole thing but wow... so nervous. What if she says the wrong thing, does the wrong thing. What if everyone can tell if she's new? What if nobody will talk to her? Do you carry a purse in a dungeon? Oh god... *dungeon*.

She didn't eat any dinner because she was too nervous to think about food and she'll probably suffer for that later but she doesn't care. The picture she has in her head refuses to go away. Tall gorgeous women in catsuits with dark lipstick and stiletto heels brandishing whips. Intimidating men in leather and chains who look her up and down and sneer because it is so obvious she's not one of *them*. What has she gotten herself into? She talks to herself, "Ilana and George are going, and they're great and normal and fine. *They* don't look like the kinky people in the movies." She thinks about calling Ilana and begging off but it's probably too late. They must be on their way by now.

She finally decides on a black dress with a slit up the leg and some high-heeled sandals. She looks at herself in the mirror. God, she wishes she were thinner. She looks like she is going to a cocktail party rather than a dungeon. The door-

37

bell rings and there is Ilana in a long black coat even though it's a warm night. "Didn't want to scare your neighbors!" she says, "You ready? You look *great!*"

"I don't know about this," says Maddie.

"Honey, I wouldn't have asked you if I didn't think you would have a good time. If you really don't want to go, then you absolutely don't have to. But I think you should give it a chance."

George is waiting in the car. He gets out to open the doors and winks at Maddie. "How're you doing?"

"I'm OK," she says. "A little nervous."

"I was terrified when I went to my first play party," he laughs. "Don't worry about it."

In the car, Ilana explains that this is a "private" party. Everyone there either belongs to a certain kinky email list or is the guest of someone who does. No one can just wander in off the street. She also runs through some of the basic "rules." There will be a social area where you can chat with people quietly. You are free to watch what is going on in the "dungeon" but don't try to talk to people who are playing. Also don't get to close to them, you don't want to invade their space or get hit with a backswing. No one will be drinking alcohol.

"I'll probably be calling George 'Master' while we're there. Don't let that throw you." George turns his eyes away from the road for a second and looks at Ilana. Some sort of current seems to pass between them suddenly and he reaches over and tousles Ilana's hair affectionately. "Good girl," he says. Ilana blushes and grins. Suddenly this quiet lawyer seems... well... Maddie can't even describe it to herself. All at once she gets how he could be "vicious" and it's thrilling.

They pull up outside what looks like a warehouse in an industrial area. "Is this it?" Maddie asks, surprised. "Yep, don't let the outside fool you."

A woman checks them in at the door and hands them some sort of disclaimer with a list of party rules. Maddie skims it and it seems to be the stuff that Ilana was telling her in the car. She scrawls her name illegibly at the bottom of the page. George hands the woman money and Maddie starts to get out her purse to pay him back. "Don't worry about it," he says, "We'd be honored to treat you to your first play party."

> **KINKY GIRL TIP**
>
> Slut cards: print up business cards with your first name or scene name and your anonymous email address to hand to hotties at a munch. Leave off the phone number, that comes later if they're lucky!
>
> **KINKY GIRL TIP**

"Oh, you're new!" says the woman who checked them in. "Welcome! Have a great time!"

They walk through another door and Maddie stops short and gasps at the sight in front of her. The place is *huge* and there are people everywhere! Not the sort of people she had pictured in her nervous fantasies, but all sorts of people. Tall, short, fat, thin, people covered with tattoos and people that look like her grandparents. They're wearing everything from shiny latex to jeans to tuxedos to nothing at all. Maddie looks down at her own dress and suddenly feels fine about it.

There's a group of people hanging out on couches sort of off to one side, and some of them wave to Ilana and George. Ilana takes off her coat and underneath she is wearing a gorgeous leather corset and a skirt. All of her curves are accentuated and her cleavage seems to go on for miles. "Could you lace me, Master?" she says to George. She braces herself against the back of a couch and he tightens the corset even more and kisses the back of her neck. She takes Maddie's hand and pulls her over to the couches, "C'mon, I want to introduce you to some folks." People stand up as they come over and shake Maddie's hand. They are all smiling and friendly, she can't get over how "normal" this all feels, even if some of them are in the most outlandish outfits.

"It's my first play party." Maddie says to one woman. "Oh god," the woman says, "I was scared out of my mind the first time! Don't worry, no one bites unless you ask them to!" Maddie looks at her, startled, and she winks, grinning.

Maddie takes a deep breath and turns towards the play area of the party. There are all sorts of pieces of equipment, some stuff she had heard of or seen pictures of and some stuff that she couldn't figure out. Ilana is at her side and she rattles off information. "That's a St. Andrew's cross, and that's a spanking bench. That's a winch, see how her has her chained to it? He can adjust it with counterweights." There is a guy tying a woman up in what looks like a spiderweb of rope. "Oh, that's John," says Ilana, "he does the most beautiful suspensions. He's a rope freak."

There's a lot of nudity and Maddie looks down, feeling somewhat embarrassed. Ilana glances at her. "Don't worry about watching," she says "They're playing in public. A lot of people actually really *like* being watched."

They walk out on the floor a bit so that Maddie can see some things closer up. There is a guy using a very long whip on someone and they give him a wide berth. He catches Ilana's eye and pauses briefly to smile at her. She gives him a thumbs-up and they move on. "That's Bill," she says, "He's *unbelievable* with a singletail. I've seen him turn lightswitches on and off." Maddie turns back and watches for a second. Bill is wielding this whip with such focus it looks like he doesn't know the rest of the world exists. There's a loud crack and the woman strapped to the cross jumps, as does Maddie. "He didn't actually hit her that time," whispers Ilana, "He was just waking her up." Maddie smiles weakly.

They come to another couple. There is a man strapped to a chair and a woman doing something that

Maddie can't quite make out. She squints and oh *God*. She's sticking needles through his nipples! Maddie turns away quickly. Ilana glances over, "Oh yeah, play-piercing. I can never watch that either," she says.

Maddie is surprised at how quickly she gets used to seeing people in various stages of undress. It also amazes her the amount of variety there is in body types. There are skinny people and people with jiggling hips and stretch marks. Very few fit the archetype she had fantasized about, those tall, perfectly formed women and broad-chested men. She starts to feel a bit more comfortable in her own skin.

They walk back over to the couches where George is talking with a group of people. As they get closer, it becomes clear that the topic of conversation is not anything kink-related but about computer networking of some sort... interspersed with the thwacking sounds and wails coming from the play area. The incongruity of it strikes Maddie as funny and she starts to laugh. Ilana rolls her eyes, "Yeah, put some geeks together and this what you get. There are crazy orgasms going on ten feet away and they're talking about *routers*. You hungry?" Maddie realizes that

> **KINKY GIRL TIP**
>
> Long-wearing lipsticks, especially the Cover Girl and Max Factor brands, stand up well to gags and long brutal kisses.
>
> **KINKY GIRL TIP**

she is, she's *starving*. There's a buffet table set up and they fill plates with chopped veggies and cheese and cookies. Ilana gets them bottles of water out of the fridge.

They sit down on the couches and talk. Ilana asks Maddie how she's feeling. "I'm really fine," she says, "Everyone's so friendly and the people that are playing seem to be doing just that, *playing*. Even the ones yelling in pain just seem to be having such a good time!"

"That's because they *are*," says Ilana, "They're doing that stuff because they really want to. Take that guy who's getting pierced. I have no desire to ever do that because I have a major thing about needles but it totally does something for him. Did you see his face? He was blissing out."

"It's really different from the movies," says Maddie.

"I know," answers Ilana, "That's exactly what I thought my first time too. There are some other sorts of parties, the really high fetish parties that might look a little more like what you were thinking of. People really use them as an opportunity to pull out all the stops with the fetishwear and there's usually not that much play going on. There's frequently a bar and dancing. They can be fun too but they're definitely different. You'll see some of this crowd at them but there are also people who just like to wear the clothes. If you want, there's one next month and we can check it out. I don't think any of my clothes will fit you but my friend Patty has a PVC dress that I bet she would lend you. Think about it."

George comes over and puts his hand on the back of Ilana's neck and whispers something in her ear. She seems to almost arch into his hand. Maddie watches, fascinated. The dynamic between them feels so powerful. They obviously love each other but there's this extra *kick* to their interactions sometimes. It just feels so open and healthy and sexy.

A big guy comes over who looks sort of like a lumberjack. Ilana leaps up and throws her arms around his neck. George laughs, "Maddie, this is Peter, the cuddliest sadist you'll ever meet."

Peter chuckles, "That's me," he says and shakes Maddie's hand. "Hey George, can I borrow this delectable morsel of a wife you somehow managed to capture? I know you guys aren't playing tonight but I'd love to turn that bouncy butt of hers pink."

Maddie is sort of shocked but when she turns to George he is smiling. "She's all yours, Pete. You did a great job last time, she couldn't sit down without squirming the whole next day."

Ilana squeezes Maddie's hand, "You OK?"

"Sure," says Maddie, "Ummm... have fun." She sits down on a couch with George and they watch Peter strap Ilana face down on a bench and start whacking her behind. Ilana squirms and giggles and Peter laughs at her.

George is smiling. "We have an agreement," he says, "If one of us doesn't feel like playing and the other one gets an offer at a party from someone we both trust and are comfortable with, then it's OK if we check in with each other. We don't play with other people when the other person isn't there. We always go home together and the sexual contact with other people is really minimal."

"Do you ever get jealous?" Maddie asks.

"I did," he says, "At the beginning. But we talked about it and came up with something that we're both totally comfortable with. Other people have different comfort levels about this sort of stuff and some people are *totally* monogamous and only play with each other. Ilana loves a good spanking and Pete is a great guy and has a hand like a sledgehammer. My hand always starts to hurt too quickly. He's totally respectful of our relationship and I have no problem with her playing with him. It also helps that I know I can say 'no' at any time and no one will be offended."

When Ilana's behind is glowing as red as a stoplight, Pete finally unstraps her and pulls her onto his lap. Maddie watches her kiss him on the cheek and then he gathers her up in his arms and carries her giggling over to George. He places her gently in George's lap, "There you go, medium-rare, just the way you like it."

George thanks him and cuddles Ilana, who is almost purring into his chest. He smiles at Maddie, "She'll be a little out of it with the endorphins for a few minutes. She bounces back pretty quickly."

Pete returns with bottles of water and hands them out. He winks at Maddie. "Anytime you want a spanking, you just let me know. I'm the best in the business."

Maddie blushes but it's hard not to like this guy. "I'll do that," she says.

Ilana stands up eventually and they start to get ready to go. They say goodbye to people and George loosens Ilana's corset for her and helps her into her coat. She turns to Maddie, "Not so bad, huh?"

"It was great," Maddie answers truthfully.

Maybe next time it will be her on that spanking bench.

Maddie's first experience with a play party was a real eye-opener for her. A lot of the images she had in her head of play parties came from the media. The reality of BDSM and what the media shows us in movies and on TV can be pretty far removed from each other. Now there are different sorts of parties, private parties, fetish parties, fetish clubs, sex parties, very small private parties in people's homes. Fetishwear parties are probably the closest to what Maddie had imagined. There's a big one in San Francisco called the Exotic Erotic Ball. Anyone can go, for a fee.

Maddie was lucky in that she had a mentor to go with. It can be easier sometimes if you have a buddy and don't have to walk in alone. Just because you go to a play party most definitely does *not* mean that you have to play. Plenty of people go to watch and to socialize. It's not like high school where the wallflowers stood around in miserable isolation. Maddie also got to see close up the interactions of one particular couple and how they dealt with issues of polyamory and play. Maddie may find out later that she wants a different arrangement for herself, but at least she started to realize the possibilities.

> ## KINKY GIRL TIP
>
> **T**ops need props too. **While** they may seem calm, cool, collected, and well, *masterful,* tops are people too and need warm fuzzies as much as anyone. If someone has just tortured you spectacularly, pull yourself out of your endorphin haze enough to tell them how fabulous they are. A nice little thank you note the next day is always tasteful and appropriate.
>
> ## KINKY GIRL TIP

Another great thing I find at play parties is the wide variety of people who attend. You find not just a vast range in body types and ages, but people from all walks of life. Conversations range from the erotic to the mundane.

What to wear depends on the party. Fetishwear is usually welcome, although if you're going to the extreme, you might want to cover up with a coat until you arrive. At some parties fetishwear is required, and you can be turned away for wearing "street clothes" or charged a higher entrance fee. Sometimes parties will

have "themes." At some parties you can wear whatever the hell you want, or nothing at all. If you're in
doubt, check with the organizers.

I've heard several accounts of people running into
coworkers, or *relatives*. After the initial shock, what
usually happens is that both parties realize they're there
for similar reasons, and while they might not choose to
chat about their shared interests at the water cooler or
at the family Christmas gathering, it's no big deal in
the larger picture.

If you're interested in public play and your partner is too, a play party can be a good choice for a first
play date. There are people around to help if something goes wrong. There also is probably a lot of equipment that you don't have at home (unless you're *very*
lucky). Generally, people bring their own toys, but the
larger pieces of bondage equipment and furniture are
in the space. There are also generally "Dungeon Moni-
tors," or DMs for short. That's not nearly as scary as it
sounds. DMs are there to make sure the rules of the
play space are being followed and everything is going
smoothly. They are also there to help if assistance is
needed.

If you're lucky enough to live somewhere that has
good parties, and you think you would like to play in
public or just go to socialize and watch, don't be scared
off by your preconceptions. They will frequently turn
out to be misconceptions. If you want, find a partner in
crime to go with and give it a shot or be brave and go it
alone. As a friend of mine says, "If it ain't going well,
fuck it, you can always just go get ice cream."

*A*s you make your way into the complex world of BDSM there are a few few decisions you will have to make – and you should make them for yourself rather than letting your dom make them for you. If you're very new at this, you may not be sure what your answers are. As you continue, the answers may change or evolve. You also may be surprised where you end up. Something you thought you wanted may be very different in reality than it was in fantasies. On the flip side, something that initially seemed abhorrent to you may become the hottest thing *ever*.

2: some important decisions

Try to keep an open mind and be aware that things change. Just because you have answered these questions once doesn't mean you shouldn't revisit them occasionally and see if they still hold true. Also, remember that these questions are just a jumping-off point as you are getting started, they by no means encompass everything you will encounter about your sexuality.

1. Are you bisexual, lesbian, or straight? Do you want to fuck girls or boys or boys who dress as girls?

Play with girls or boys? Many women play with other women but don't have sex with them. Maddie and Suki both explore this issue in this book and come to very different conclusions. A common misperception is that as a woman in the scene, you have to be bisexual. Nope, you can fuck whoever you want. Also keep in mind that gender can be fluid. You may find people who are transsexual, transvestite, or transgendered to be your ideal partners. Does that mean you're ummmm... gay or straight? Does it really matter what you call yourself if you're doing who you want to be doing? There may not be an easy label to slap onto your forehead so don't worry about it.

2. Are you polyamorous or monogamous? Or somewhere in between? I am not going to get too deeply into issues of polyamory because you could write an entire book about it. In fact, people have: see the suggested reading list in the back. Basically, do you want one partner or more than one? Some people in the scene who call themselves monogamous in the BDSM world would be considered poly in the "vanilla" world. Some people play with a few people but only fuck one. Some people fuck a few people but only play with one. Some people fuck a lot of people and play with a lot of people. Some people fuck and play with only one person. You get the picture? There are endless variants and it can take time to figure out where you fit into the spectrum. It can also take some trial and error. Approach it with honesty and a lot of communication with your partners.

3. Are you interested in play that's about sensation, or about control, or a combo? Some people use S/M to mean the first kind and D/S to mean the second kind. S/M stands for sadomasochism. Some people are purely into this for the sensation of giving or receiving pain or other sensations, and have very little interest in power dynamic: smack my bottom but if you call me your slave I will kick your ass. A lot of folks refer to one person in such scenes as the top and the other person as the bottom. (In other communities, top and bottom are catchall terms meaning the person-in-charge and the person-not-in-charge, so don't assume that your terms mean the same thing as the next guy's terms, particularly if you're playing with folks you don't know.)

D/S, which stands for dominance and submission, involves a power exchange dynamic of some sort. You have a dominant and a submissive (again, some people use dominant and submissive as *their* catchall terms – I know, this is all confusing).

Many people are into versatility. Many people (called switches) like to switch roles, sometimes they like to be on the bottom and sometimes the top. Confusing? Hell yeah. It will become clearer as time goes on.

4. What kinds of play do you want to do right away, and what kinds might you want to try someday with the right partner if the situation presents itself, and what kinds do you think you want to keep away from? There are probably more kinds of play than you've ever imagined. If you're new to all this, I strongly recom-

mend that you go get one of the good basic guidebooks in the back of this book and read it through carefully. Would you want to try splosh? Scat? Would you like to have a sissy maid or a puppy? Do you have a clue what any of those terms mean, and, if not, how will you find out? And what will you do about your own safety and limits – will you, for example, do any sort of play that involves blood or the piercing of the skin (cuttings, needle-play)?

5. Do you want to try edgy play or would you rather stay on the more conservative side of things? Remember what is edgy for you may be old hat for someone else. What you think is no big deal may make their head spin. There seems to be sort of a hierarchy to BDSM activities. Stuff like spanking or flogging or nipple clamps is at one end. Stuff like piercing, suspensions and branding is at the other end. There's a hell of a lot of stuff in the middle. It's not school, you don't have to graduate from one grade of BDSM and progress automatically to the next. Find what you're comfortable with. If something really doesn't appeal to you, you certainly don't have to try it. Nobody gets to make fun of you or act like you're not a good bottom or top because you don't want to try something, and you should never ever play with someone who tries to pull that kind of mindgame on you. Figure out your limits and be firm about them.

6. How much do you want to incorporate BDSM into your life? Do you want it to be a 24/7 arrangement

or do you just want it in the bedroom? Or do you just want to go get your ass beaten once a month? Once a year? A lot of BDSM erotica deals with 24/7 relationships. That means there is a power exchange dynamic in a relationship 24 hours a day, seven days a week. That may seem like the hottest thing in the world to you but in reality it involves a lot of work. You may find that seven days a week is too much for you but the occasional weekend is fun. You may just want a D/S dynamic in the bedroom. You might just have the occasional itch for it. Fantasy and reality can be very different things.

A special note on collars and other relationship symbols. I tend to take these fairly seriously. A good decision to make is to think about what a collar means to you. It can just be a piece of jewelry: you can now buy them at teenybopper accessory stores at the mall. Some people have play collars that they just use during the scene. Sometimes it can be symbolic of a more serious D/S relationship. Alternatives to something that looks like it should be on a Rottweiler are anklets or other pieces of jewelry, piercings, brandings, and tattoos – but remember, the further down that list you get, the harder they are to get rid of; even laser surgery leaves a scar.

7. Do you want to play in public or does the thought of being beaten or beating someone in front of an audience give you the willies? Just because you're kinky doesn't mean you have to go play at parties. You may

find your interactions are hotter when you're alone with your partner. You may totally get off on being watched, or watching other people. There may be certain activities you like doing in public and others that you want to do at home. Some people play at parties but reserve the fucking for the bedroom, or the kitchen floor, or whatever. Other people happily go at it in the middle of a crowded dungeon.

8. This is a really important one. What are your safer sex standards? Do you require a barrier for all sexual activity? Dental dams for cunnilingus? Will you blow someone without a condom? Does someone have to wear a glove when they finger you? Do you use condoms with your secondary partners but have unprotected sex with your primary partner? Condoms for anal sex but bareback for vaginal intercourse? Do you have a death wish and fuck everybody without a condom? Educate yourself about disease transmission and evaluate the level of risk you want to take. Be very honest with your partners about any STDs you may have and ask them about theirs.

You may be cross-eyed by the end of this section. Who knew there were so many choices? You just wanted to get a little spanking! Remember, these are a jumping-off point. Some of them may apply to you and some may not. It helps to at least have an idea of what some of your choices are. When I went to graduate school, the most important thing I learned was how much I _didn't_ know. Exploring your sexuality can be a lot like that.

*M*addie knows she shouldn't go to Dallas. She's new at all this, and nobody's ever told her "the rules" about safely meeting strangers for the first time. But she's pretty sure that flying to Texas to have sex – no, not just sex, but intense, kinky, submissive, you-got-me-where-you-want-me-baby-now-take-me-down-*hard* sex – with a man you've only met on a computer screen and a telephone receiver is not the act of a sensible young woman.

But she *wants* to go. Every nerve of her newly awakened

*she looks out the **window** of the plane as it descends into dallas...*

sexuality is throbbing with anticipation. A portion of her anatomy about one-half square inch and weighing about an ounce, located squarely between her thighs, has taken complete control of about one hundred forty pounds of highly intelligent, functional, twenty-four-year-old female.

... She had met him online. She was shiny sparkling new, aflame with the discovery of a whole kinky world out there. She was a star student in a small

KINKY GIRL TIP

How to explain the crazy noises emanating from your apartment to the neighbors? "I have a poltergeist." There's really no answer for that one.

KINKY GIRL TIP

school in the Deep South with no local kink community, no rational people to tell her how crazy the idea was, how utterly unreasonable. Would she have listened to them anyway?

He talked to her on the phone every morning and evening, gave her tasks to perform, sent her a collar to wear while she slept, told her how he wanted to use her and fuck her, while she listened and touched herself. She moaned into the receiver when she came.

Weeks went by. She was wet all the time. One day he told her that he *needed* her to come to Dallas for a few days. Her answer started at her groin and leapt directly through her lips, coming nowhere near her brain.

She didn't know his last name or have his home address. He wanted her to step off that cliff without a safety net. "The leap of trust," he called it. Insanity, she knew it to be, and didn't care at all.

She bought the ticket and spent the intervening time wallowing in anticipation and doubt. She knew this was crazy, *knew* it. But it didn't matter. The thing seemed to take on a life of its own. She was going, it seemed inevitable.

She tries to read on the plane but can't focus. Her mind keeps jumping from the story on the page to the vivid movies in her head. What's happening to *her* is infinitely more interesting than what's going on in the book.

She has told no one she's going. By the time she boards the plane she is already wet and trembling.

She chews gum and stares out the window. The trip is only about four hours long but it feels like days are passing. Before the plane lands, she goes to the restroom to check her makeup and hair, to refresh her perfume. As she reapplies her eyeliner, she tries to see herself objectively in the mirror. Does she *look* like a submissive? Does she capture that ineffable quality of... what? She lowers her head and peers up from under her lashes. Her clit flutters like a captive bird.

Is this particular shade of lipstick really appropriate for a submissive – or maybe something with a little more rose in it? Maybe submissives ought to look a little more, well, *demure*? She wipes off the offensive red and applies the pinkish rose, thankful that she remembered to bring it. The plane runs over

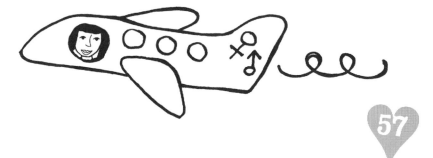

a bump in the sky, her hand slips and she wipes it off again, starting over with her trembling fingers, struggling for control of her hands, her mouth.

In Dallas he picks her up at the gate but doesn't say anything after "Hello." She trails mutely behind him, carrying her own bags because he has not offered. She is sure anyone in the airport, watching them, can tell what is going on. He has not allowed her to orgasm for a week before her visit. She had only cheated once and felt guilty about it but the orgasm had been remarkably powerful. Surely unresolved sexual tension hangs between them in a visible cloud.

The tile of the motel bathroom floor is cold underneath her. She is bound tightly, wrist to ankle, gagged and hooded at his feet. He puts a hand on the back of her head and she starts.

"You're mine now. I can do anything I want to you and nobody knows where you are."

The awareness of this truth washes over her like a wave. It is the most erotic moment of her life.

... She spent the weekend with him in that innocuous motel room, utterly vulnerable and utterly aroused the entire time.

He was thirty years older than she was and his skin felt crepey under her fingertips, like a plum well on its way to rot. She felt disloyal for noticing.

She returned to her life. He turned whiney and

unreasonable after the trip, demanding that she leave school and return to him. Reason and logic edged back in through the doors of her psyche as he got more petulant. She knew his name now. One day she was quite simply done.

About four years later, she read a news story about a man who called himself "Slavetrainer" online and lured submissive women to his property in Kansas City. He held them prisoner until he was finished, and then, sometimes, he murdered them. Several bodies were found in oil drums around his land. The papers all asked the same question, "What were these women thinking? How could they be so appallingly naive?" She remembered the hand pressing down the back of her head. Maddie knew exactly what they were (or weren't) thinking.

I can't tell you never to succumb to sexual idiocy: maybe you will, and maybe you won't. Maddie did, and survived it; I have, and survived it; "Slavetrainer's" victims did, and some of them survived it, and some of them didn't.

Women talk about men disparagingly, saying that they are thinking with their little heads or joking about blood being diverted from their brains to their cocks. What is rarely mentioned is that there is an equivalent phenomenon for women. At least, there is for me, and I have certainly seen other women,

59

usually intelligent and clear-thinking, basically turn into insane people when they're really, really turned on by someone or some situation.

Maddie thought her Dallas escapade was hideously embarrassing, that no one else could possibly be so *stupid*, until she heard a friend's story. Hers involved meeting a dom on the Internet, buying a ticket, and flying to *Tokyo* three days later. He fucked her exclusively up the ass and had a penchant for doing it in alleyways. She ended up just fine also. In the annals of sexual idiocy, Tokyo trumps Dallas any day.

I like to refer to it as thinking with my clit and it can be dangerous and dump me in the middle of risky situations that I would never have gone *near* if I weren't so damn turned on. I'm not saying *don't* think with your clit. Succumbing to sexual idiocy can lead one (occasionally) to erotic nirvana. But know your risks and educate yourself about how to live out your fantasies in the safest and sanest way possible.

If you fly to Dallas to meet a stranger, you could be killed. You may do it anyway. You may feast on that knowledge. I hope you won't, because you can have ninety-five percent of the fun and five percent of the risk by using a safecall – remember what I said about safecalls earlier in the book? A couple of "Slavetrainer's" would-be victims used this strategy, and are alive to tell the tale.

Make your partner accountable to a third person for your whereabouts and safe return. You can be as thorough as you choose to be. If the person is as concerned about your well-being as he should be, he will cooperate. If he refuses to cooperate, assume that he has something to hide, and that this is probably not someone with whom you want to spend time.

However, if he really wants to deceive you, he probably still can. Be aware that you are taking a risk.

The fact is that some of us are turned on to danger. If this is you, read this next part carefully.

When you play with dangerous toys because they turn you on, you risk getting hurt. (Duh.) The average person is more likely to get struck by lightning than stabbed on a normal day. However, if you are a knifeplay aficionado, your risk of being stabbed increases exponentially. You may like the risk, but you don't like the reality: chances are you don't particularly want to be stabbed. Playing with knives can be very hot because it *is* dangerous, they inspire fear for a reason. But a trip to the hospital wouldn't be nearly as hot.

So educate yourself about knifeplay if that's your kink. Go to classes. Play with people who have a reputation in the kink community for being good with knives. Learn enough about knifeplay to be able to tell if your partner is skilled. There will still be risks to knifeplay, there could be an earthquake in the middle of a scene. But you can mitigate the risk, not succumb to sexual idiocy, and maintain the erotic edge.

I like to play with fear, danger, and the unknown. These days, away from that first heady rush of sexual awakening, I try to mitigate the risks. One person I play with, knowing I like some fear, told me that he actually *was* dangerous. I knew the story he referred to. He had tied someone to a St. Andrew's cross without anchoring it to the floor, and it had tipped over and fractured her wrist. He didn't understand that crossed the line from good fear into just scary not-turned-on fear. He managed to lose the erotic edge by getting *too* real and scary. I had no desire to fracture my wrist or any other bone in my body. It's a fine line in both directions. One can become too predictable or too unpredictable.

Real safety lies in abstinence. Barring that as being completely unreasonable (well, for anyone who's reading this book, anyway), educate yourself about the risks you're taking. Be aware if you're blinded by lust. Take risks if risks are what you like, but take them *consciously*.

KINKY GIRL TIP

Dietary precautions. Drinking soda while wearing a corset is an interesting experience. Always pee before getting tied up. Don't eat really spicy food the night before anal play. Indian food and buttplugs are a nasty combo.

KINKY GIRL TIP

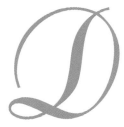

Dear Maddie,

So I've read all the books and taken all the workshops on negotiation, and filled out all the damn checklists until my fucking pencil is worn to a nubbin, and a fat lot of good it's done me. I'm writing this on my laptop lying in bed surrounded by a sea of used Kleenex because I've spent the last, oh, seven or eight hours crying. I'm not sure I'm ever going to top again. This sucks. But I suppose I should begin at the beginning, huh?

As you know, John and I have been playing for a couple of months now, and it's been going pretty well – a couple of stumbles, but most of the scenes have been good and one or two really hot ones (that butt of

> *"his face **convulsed** into an expression i can't **begin** to describe..."*

his is to die for) – we haven't quite said the l-word yet but I know we've both been thinking it (well, at least *I* have). And one of the things he's been asking for is to explore what he calls "the girl thing" – he's really wanted to cross-dress, fantasized about it for years. We've talked it out during our other play – you know, I've called those awful dingy tighty-whities of his, the kind they all wear, his "panties," stuff like that – but we've never actually done anything like that – and he's admitted to finding the idea a little bit scary but really really *really* a turnon – and we'd finally decided to go ahead and try it.

I spent weeks buying up stuff. John's not a small guy, and you don't find ruffled blouses in size 32 to fit my budget just anywhere. Most of it I got at Goodwill and places like that, which I tell you wasn't easy (although it was a lot of fun – especially the looks I got, or imagined I got, from the little old ladies behind the counter). Some from regular stores. One or two I had to send away for – you just don't find red patent-leather pumps in size 13 anywhere in this town. But I did luck out on a big box of makeup in every color imaginable at Walgreens for just $9.99 – at last, a use for all those make-up tips I'd gone on reading in all the women's magazines all those years even though I've done my own face the exact same way since my 24th birthday. Altogether, I had to have spent over twelve hours and a couple of hundred bucks putting that outfit together, and that doesn't even count the time I spent jilling off thinking about what he was going to look like in it and what I was going to do to him once he was dressed up in all of it – the nice thing, I thought, about a crossdressed guy was going to be that it was going to be

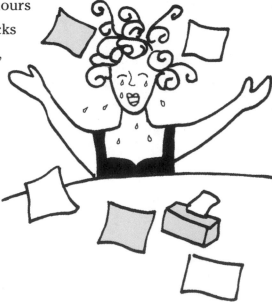

the best things about getting to play with a girl without actually having to confront an honest-to-god pussy, which always
freak me out just a teeny bit, you know?

So I finally had a pretty good outfit together: the ruffled
blouse (cream-colored polyester), bra, panties, garter belt,
hose, black mini, red heels, belt, earrings, a bunch of bangles
so he'd hear himself jingle every time he moved. No wig,
but he wears his hair on the long side and I decided that
with a touch of the curling iron, a hefty shot of Aquanet and
a lot of willing suspension of disbelief we'd get by OK. So I
called him to set up a date, and we wound up having a pretty
hot phone sex session just talking about "Jolene" and what
she was going to look like in her pretty new clothes. Ah, the
power of the imagination. That, and hubris. Shit, now I'm
starting to get weepy again. Just a sec...

OK, better now. So the day came and I went over to
his place. I set up a comfortable couple of chairs, some-
place where there were no mirrors – I didn't want him to
see "Jolene" until she was completely finished. I think I
spent more time putting him together than I did on myself the night of my junior prom – it had to be two or
three hours, anyway. I shaved his face so close it glowed
pink afterward, tweezed his eyebrows, curled every hair
on his head. Perfumed, powdered, painted his nails rosy
pink, put on at least four coats of mascara (ever tried to
put mascara on someone who's never worn it before?).
Stuffed that bra with enough Kleenex to sop up a
theaterful of "Terms of Endearment"-watchers – that boy
was *stacked*. And, by the time I was done, there was

Jolene – not passable exactly, but, well, I guess you'd have to call him pretty. I felt like Pygmalion falling in love with my own creation.

I took "her" hand, held my other hand gently over her eyes (no messing up the eye makeup!), led her to the full-length mirror on the master bedroom closet. "OK, you ready?" I asked.

"Ready," she said. She seemed to be trembling at a frequency slightly too high for the human eye to perceive.

"John, meet Jolene," I said, and dropped my hand.

Maddie, there is no way I could have been ready for what happened next. There was a long, still moment as John looked at himself – herself – in the mirror. He took a step backward. He began to breathe audibly and fast. His face convulsed into an expression I can't begin to describe – something like a trapped animal, with his lips pulled back over his teeth in a snarl, his pupils contracted, his eyebrows high and drawn together. He turned toward me and I shrank back – for a fraction of a moment I thought he was going to hit me. Then he turned and ran from the room.

I stood there for what must have been a couple of minutes, frozen, utterly unsure what had just happened and even more unsure what to do about it. Then, slowly, I followed him. He was standing naked in the middle of the living room, breathing like he'd just finished a marathon. The clothes were scattered all over the place – he'd obviously thrown them with some force, and a couple of garments were torn. His lipstick was smeared all the way across his face to one ear, and a matching smear showed on the back of his

hand where he'd obvi-
ously tried to wipe it off
himself. He looked at me,
still breathing hard, and
did not say a word.

> **KINKY GIRL TIP**
>
> Bad breath and BO are their own particular form of torture. Some people like the smell of good honest *clean* sweat but bring your Listerine pocket packs and stay kissably fresh.
>
> **KINKY GIRL TIP**

I thought fast about
what to do. I could, of
course, simply go – prob-
ably the safest course of
action. But I'd played a
part in getting him into
this state of mind, and I felt like I had some responsibility
to help him calm down enough to figure out what had gone
so wrong. "Do you want to talk about it?" I asked. "Are you
calm enough to sit down for a minute?"

Thank heavens, that seemed to be the right tack; his
eyes focused a bit and his breathing slowed. "Just give me
a second to pull myself together," he said in a grating voice.
I nodded. We stood there for another minute or two. Finally,
he closed his eyes, gave a visible little shake – like a dog
shaking off water – and sat down on the couch.

I sat down next to him and, cautiously, took his hand.
"I'll just sit here with you," I offered. "You can talk when
you feel ready."

We just sat like that for a long time, maybe twenty minutes. Finally, he began to talk. He didn't know what had
triggered the freakout... he'd just looked at himself in the
mirror, seen someone he didn't know, felt humiliated and
furious and terrified, and completely lost his self-control –

had to leave the room before he'd done violence to me.

We sat like that and I let him talk, offered what reassurance I could. I had a strong sense of having dodged a bullet – I think he'd come closer than even he realized to having really lost it badly, badly enough to really hurt me.

Finally, he'd talked himself out. I hugged him, helped him wash off the last of the make-up, tucked him into bed, let myself out, climbed into my car – and burst into uncontrollable tears. I cried so hard I couldn't think of starting the car up and driving home for at least fifteen minutes, and then when I finally pulled myself together enough to drive the few minutes back to my apartment, I got home, started crying again, cried all the way through making myself a cup of tea, and I've been crying ever since.

All those people who think bottoming is scary – they don't *know*. Bottoming may have its scary moments, but I have a hard time believing it could get much scarier or more hurtful than this. I don't know if John and I will ever be the same again. Hell, I don't know if *I'll* ever be the same again. It'll be a long time before I buy any guy another garter belt, I do know that.

Your tired and tearful friend,
Suki

Sometimes the best-planned scene can derail completely and leave you wondering what the hell just happened and how do you make it right? Sometimes nobody is at fault and all you can do is figure out the best way to pick up the pieces.

BDSM is powerful stuff and can trigger powerful emotions, even emotions you never expected. Sometimes repressed memories rear their ugly little heads at precisely the wrong moment. Sometimes stuff comes to the surface gradually after a scene. I once felt sort of bad during a scene but couldn't figure out why. It wasn't until the next morning that I connected the dots and concluded that some bad memories had come up for me. I didn't like the emotional fallout and chose not to do that sort of play again.

Suki and John hit it head-on. Something came up for him during the experience, something that neither of them had expected and certainly not something they had fantasized about. No one made a mistake, they had planned, negotiated, communicated. It just went wrong. I'm not a therapist, I don't know why. Apparently neither did John or Suki.

So what do you do if your bottom freaks out on you? Basically, you do exactly what Suki did. If they're bound, you get them the hell out. Then you try to figure out what is going on, preferably not from a "I'm your dom, tell me what is going on" kind of space but from a nurturing caring space. They may not be able to tell you and you can only offer whatever comfort they want. Caring and compassion, the two "C's." Another good idea is to try to revisit it when everything has calmed down and emotions aren't quite so raw and see if you can make some sense of things.

You do have a responsibility here. Even if you didn't do anything wrong, you're in this together and you can't cut and run when things take a decided turn for the unsexy. If you're just in this for the hot sex and can't deal with emotions, you're playing the wrong game.

If you're the bottom and the freaker-outer (freakee?), basketcase, whatever, communicate the best you can. Some knee-jerk anger towards the top may come up even if it wasn't their fault. Try to contain that and reason your way through it. Remember, your top is probably just as upset as you are, if not more. Poor Suki was an emotional wreck. Tops need aftercare too, especially in this sort of situation. They make themselves very vulnerable by taking on responsibility. Even when scenes go well, there is a common phenomenon dubbed "top drop" – sadness, depression, just generally feeling low after a scene. When a scene goes badly like this one, it can be devastating for a top.

What could Suki and John have done better? Maybe they could have gone at it a little more slowly... not the whole shebang at once. Other than that, they did the best they could and things went badly. Unfortunately, life is sometimes like that. Kinky sex is no exception.

*M*addie had fucked him years ago when they were both home from college. The sex itself had been unremarkable but kind of hot – just because it *was* so blatantly casual.

Years later, she finds herself back in his bed. A few beers, some conversation, a familiar kiss, an invitation and there she is. He doesn't know she is kinky and she doesn't feel the need to tell him. She would dip a toe in the vanilla pool for old times' sake. She doesn't feel like talking about it and answering all

back in his bed: "i thought you liked that kinky shit"...

the inevitable questions. Just some nice, old-fashioned, uncomplicated fucking. It used to be so simple.

He smells the same. It's an uncomplicated scent as well and she likes it. Ivory soap and shaving cream. No cologne. A little bit of clean sweat. It reminds her of being younger. His body is different, a little thicker and some more fur. She runs her fingers through it and smiles. His cock is small,

71

she had forgotten, but even that is somehow endearing. He uses it well and she settles into the rhythm of his thrusts.

Suddenly pain, completely unexpected, blossoms across her upper chest and she screams.

"What the *fuck*???"

He rears up, surprised by her reaction but looking absurdly pleased with himself at the same time.

"I thought you liked that kinky shit." Apparently someone had been talking, or he had looked at the tattoos and piercings and drawn his own conclusions.

He has bitten her *hard*. She massages the angry indentations his teeth have left and feels the aching of the bruising beginning underneath.

She pushes him off and grabs her clothes, pulling them on as she leaves. The bruises left by his teeth last for two weeks.

That incident left Maddie wary of vanilla men. Similar incidences in my own life have done the same to me: too often, vanilla men just don't "get it."

The assumption that random pain and violence is acceptable scares me and makes me feel vulnerable. Images from the media have built up frightening and dangerous portrayals of BDSM and vanilla men seem like they hear the words without understanding the music. They don't know the protocols of etiquette that I am used to, and I have the sense that they're waiting for me to act my role in a play to which I haven't been handed the script.

Perverts, for all their oddities, can be predictable. They have the same set of maps in their glovebox. They run on the commonly accepted principles of safe, sane and consensual. Very rarely do the media images make that clear.

The people with the most dangerous toys can be the safest.

I feel like I've lost the knack of vanilla dating because I have become so used to the maps of the BDSM world. We become very good at laying our cards on the table.

I went out on a "vanilla" date recently, with a perfectly nice and attractive man. It was pleasant but rather baffling. I felt completely clueless by the end of it. It had none of the signposts that I was familiar with. As we said goodbye, I had no idea if the guy even liked me. We had talked about inconsequential things. He hadn't asked if I fuck in public or if I liked bondage. The logical conclusion of a date for me was an invitation to play. This one ended with a rather gentle kiss. I was stymied. I felt adrift in the vanilla dating world. I didn't go out with him again.

addie isn't "out" to her family. It just never really seemed necessary. Maybe there were moments, in the first heady flush of the discovery process, when she wanted to confess her newfound sexuality. It felt so *important*, like something that should be shared and celebrated. Fortunately, she made it through that giddy period without making that particular mistake.

The reality of the matter is that her parents are older and relatively sexually conservative. Hell... *very* sexually conservative. Her mother in particular: during one conversation, her mother actually told her

*"you got some **mail** in a plain brown envelope," he said casually...*

that she thought blowjobs were perverted, that she had never done that and she was sure none of her friends had either. Maddie remembers feeling distinctly sorry for her father. The revelation of her own activities would be a matter of horror. It would be a selfish confession rather than a cause for celebration. There isn't really much deception involved: she hasn't lived at home since she was a teenager.

Maddie goes home to visit. Her father picks her up at the airport. Her mother is away, coming home the next evening. Maddie's making sandwiches with her dad in the kitchen.

"You got some mail," he says offhandedly.

"Uh-huh," she mutters while trying to decide which kind of jam to have on her sandwich. Her mother makes a quince jelly which is exquisite.

"It was in a plain brown envelope so your mother opened it. She didn't know if it was important."

Uh-oh. Little tiny alarm bells start to ring in her head. Plain brown envelope? Nothing innocent comes in a plain brown envelope.

"It was from a place called The Branding Iron."

Suddenly it felt like her stomach had fallen straight out of her vagina and onto the floor. *The Branding Iron??!!* The Branding Iron wasn't some fluffy little woman-oriented vibrator company. The Branding Iron sold *everything*. It catered to the most hard-core perverts out there and had everything from electric buttplugs to... oh *god*... the tinny little alarm bells in her head had changed to full-on screaming sirens.

"The Branding Iron? As in cows?" Oh no...where the hell had that come from? She wondered. *Cows?* Act nonchalant... don't drop the bottle you're holding.

He continues, "It had stuff like dildos and nipple clamps and..."

She misses the rest of the sentence as she starts to go into shock from hearing her father utter the words "nipple clamps." This is the stuff nightmares are made of... this is *exactly* why she never gives her parents' address out to anyone even *remotely* kinky.

"It really upset your mother. She kept saying 'Look what your daughter has gotten into!'"

Maddie laughs, hoping it doesn't sound strained. "I wish my life was that interesting. I can't even get laid." That's it... throw him off by cracking jokes. "I wonder what I ordered to get on *that* mailing list?" she says, remembering an uncomfortably large black buttplug that one top had expressly commanded that she purchase.

"You had better call them and get off their list. Another one came and I threw it away before your mother saw it."

"Oh believe me," she says fervently. "I will be getting off of that list."

She waits until he goes to bed and then calls the company and gets an unlucky young man on the phone.

"You sent your catalogue to me at *my parents' address*!" she hisses into the phone. "And my 70-year-old *mother* opened it! What are you guys *thinking?*"

> **KINKY GIRL TIP**
> Bikinis don't cover much. If you're planning to go to the beach the next day, you might want to mention that to your whip-wielding partner in advance.
> **KINKY GIRL TIP**

"Oh my God," he stammers. "I'm so sorry... I'll take you off the list right away... and please apologize to your mother."

"I will never, *never* speak of this with my mother."

And she never did.

Moral of the story: beware of the National Address Forwarding service.

♥

So who do you come out to? You've discovered this wonderful part of your sexuality and you want to share it. Remember that's what is done cannot be undone. It's tough to tell someone and then take it back ("Oh, *that?* You thought I was *serious* about that??!")

Make your choices carefully. This country is very conservative when it comes to alternative sexuality for the most part and you may get some negative reactions. You may also have to deal with a lot of misperceptions put forward about BDSM in popular culture. Very rarely is kink portrayed in a positive or realistic way: think *Pulp Fiction*. If you have children, do you think they're equipped to understand your sexuality? I have also heard of kink being used against people in child custody cases, and I personally know a few people who have lost their jobs when their kink has come to the attention of their employers. These are all things to take into account when you make your decisions. Be prepared for confusion, questions, maybe embarrassment. If you get lucky, people may be happy for you. If you're not so lucky, they may never speak to you again.

My personal rule of thumb is that I don't come out to people I wouldn't normally speak about my sex life with. That is the level that I am comfortable with. What you're comfortable with may differ. The relationship I have with my parents does not involve speaking about sexuality, mine or theirs. That may change after the publication of this book. (Hi Mom!) The relationship I have with many of my friends does involve talking about sexuality. Most of my friends know I'm kinky. Many of my friends are kinky themselves. I have chosen not to come out in the workplace. If someone asks about my weekend I smile and enjoy the naughty little secret of that fabulous scene on Saturday night. I always make sure not to get marks that can't be covered with clothing.

One of the best experiences I had coming out involved one of my closest girlfriends who I had known since childhood. I agonized a bit about telling her and then finally just did it. "Oh my god!" she said, "Peter and I have been doing that stuff for years and I was afraid to tell *you!*" I came out to another friend and she said she had always wanted to ask her boyfriend to spank her and knowing I was kinky gave her the chutzpah to do it.

Some people are out all over the place and have no problem with that. If that works in their lives then it's great. You have to look at your own circumstances, how you feel, and the people around you and make your own decisions. Not choosing to tell the neighbors that you like puppy play does not mean you are ashamed. You're just being discreet and setting boundaries around your privacy. You get to decide how "out" you want to be. But, as a friend of mine says, "Once that toothpaste is out of the tube, there's no fucking way to put it back in!"

Once you've made your decisions, there are some ways to protect your privacy should you care to. Many people in the scene use pseud-onyms. When someone stands up at a munch and introduces himself as Master Ravenclaw, it's a pretty safe bet it doesn't say that on his birth certificate. Many people seem to have a predilection for animal names, Wolf, Bear, Raven. Strangely enough, I have yet to run into someone proudly calling him-self Guinea Pig or Penguin.

No matter how proud you are of that beautiful black leather collar with the shiny studs and the big heavy pad-lock that your Master bestowed on you, if you don't want to come out to your family, you may not want to wear it home for Thanksgiving. No, they won't think it's a necklace. I promise.

If you're going to join kinky mailing lists, you may not want to use your work email address – there are many anony-mous email services, like Yahoo. Surfing a lot of kinky sites at work may also not be the best idea – in fact, it can get you fired from many companies. If you are going to get kinky catalogues sent to you or other kink-related mail, think about getting a post office box or private mailbox. Most BDSM or-ganizations are very attuned to people's desires for privacy and allow you to sign up under any name you wish. Quick note: remember which name you used. I once walked into a party and couldn't remember which name I had on the list and had to stand there giving them all the options, "Ummmm...try this. Nope? Ok, um what about this one. No? Hmmmm... maybe my porn star name?"

One thing I have discovered is that the desire for pri-vacy seems to vary depending on what part of the country you're in. On the East Coast, people seemed to be very care-ful with their identities. In liberal San Francisco, at one of the first events I attended, someone handed me his actual business card, name of the company, phone number, the works. I was shocked. He was fine with his information being out there and it didn't worry him.

If you run into someone on the street that you saw last weekend getting the crap beaten out of them in a club, it's generally not a good idea to walk up and say "Hey! Great scene, Wolf! You were howling like an *animal!* How are those welts?" Respect their privacy. They may approach you, they may be out to the people they're with, or if they're alone they may be happy to talk about it. But if you happen to say that in front of their 70-year-old grandmother, or kid, or coworker, or vanilla friend, then you've taken away their right to set up their own boundaries of disclosure. If you don't know how out someone is and you run into them in public, the safe bet is to smile and walk on by. We perverts need some sort of signal we can flash at each other like a secret club. If there is one, I haven't learned it yet.

> **KINKY GIRL TIP**
>
> Here's a tip you won't get anywhere else (except from a pissed-off top who's trying to clean his favorite toy): Glitter is pretty and fun and girly. Do *not* adorn yourself with glitter if you're planning to play. It gets all over toys and all over your partner and infuriates even the most patient top. Most tops don't appreciate being all sparkly for days after a scene. Silly of them, I know, but trust me on this, I learned the hard way.
>
> **KINKY GIRL TIP**

Keep in mind, there are public events and private events. Some play parties are private and people can only come if they are on a list or belong to an organization or are somehow invited. As a general rule, cameras are not allowed at these events. There are public clubs and events that anyone can come to, provided they are over eighteen. Every so often, news reporters do an "expose" on sex clubs in San Francisco and smuggle cameras in duffle bags and show blurry pictures with cruddy lighting. At any event you go to, you may run into someone you know from your "vanilla" life. Chances are, they will be just as concerned with their privacy as you are with yours. There are some very public events like Folsom Street Fair in San Francisco. It's a great event, but there are media cameras there and if you don't want to risk your face showing up on the five o'clock news, you may want to either not show up or wear some really big sunglasses.

If you are extremely concerned about your privacy, you may decide that public play or socializing in the BDSM community is not something you're interested in. As long as you're being safe, there's nothing that says private play can't be hot.

*M*en seem to swarm around new submissives like flies. Women who have been around for a while stand back and make snide comments about "vultures" and "new meat." Maddie never understood the fascination with "newbies" until she tasted that particular fruit herself.

Bill shows up at a munch. Young, attractive, well-spoken, respectful. He asks if they can meet for coffee and she agrees.

He has all sorts of questions about the scene. He is fascinated by everything and encourages her to talk... to tell him about scene dynamics,

*she didn't usually **top**, but she saw **something** in his eyes...*

about play, about her experiences. It makes her feel... well... interesting.

"Why did you come to that munch?" she asks him.

"Well," he answers thoughtfully. "My friend Sasha told me about it. I'd always had these fantasies but my ex never wanted to try anything. She thought it was weird. I dunno...." He gets a faraway look in his eyes. "I just thought maybe there might be someone out there who would try some things with me. I've thought about them for so long but I'm from the Midwest, just moved here three months ago. Believe me, no one back there would think this sort of stuff is any way all right." Apparently his ex-girlfriend not only didn't want to try anything, she told him that such stuff was "warped" and suggested he see a psychiatrist.

Maddie smiles at him. "You're in San Francisco now. Nothing is too weird. There are probably plenty of people who would be more than happy to play with you."

He is hanging on her every word. So eager... it was sweet.

Later, he takes her out to dinner. Things progress nicely and they end up going to his place and playing. He wants to be tied up so she blindfolds him and ties him to his bed. She uses her nails and her teeth. Just a little, just a taste. He is so hard it is amazing and he moans underneath her, arching his body up to meet her. She tops him, something she doesn't do very often but he wants so badly to experience it.

> **KINKY GIRL TIP**
>
> Fuck Atkins, carbs are good. A woman brought me a gorgeous big dark truffle once after a particularly heavy scene and I deified her on the spot.
>
> **KINKY GIRL TIP**

She whispers in his ear, "Do you like that? Look how hard you are...look how turned on..." She bites his nipple, not too hard, and he yelps softly. "Awww....does that hurt? Didn't hurt *me* at all." She scrapes her nails across his balls and he seems to strain towards her and pull away all at once. She pulls the blindfold off him so that she can see his eyes. It is like being with a kid at Christmas. He is so eager that her slightest touch makes him absolutely cross-eyed with lust and it is intoxicating to her. Everything is new to him... everything she does is like magic. She feels so powerful.

Suddenly she gets it. *This* is why they want the new girls. They want to see that look on their faces when everything is new. They want to be Santa Claus.

Maddie only played with Bill the one time, but the experience stayed with her for weeks. Fantasies and activities that she thought she'd been bored with suddenly seemed fresh, hot, sexy again – somehow, topping a novice had made her feel almost like a novice again herself, with that same sense of possibility, that same openmouthed excitement.

What she'd done to Bill was lightweight compared to scenes she'd done with her own tops but it had blown his mind. It's *fun* to blow someone's mind.

Some tops have admitted that they are intimidated by the idea of playing with me because I'm more experienced than they are. They don't want to see judgment in my eyes, or imagined (or not-so-imagined) criticism.

What I usually try to explain (with varying success) is that for me, physical skill with toys can be learned, that can come later. What really gets me going is the look in someone's eyes, the tone in their voice. They can have no toys at all, they don't even have to touch me to make me wet.

Some people just aren't that great at it. Usually it's because they're trying too hard and not listening to the signals they're receiving from their partner. I feel especially critical when the top seems to be operating off some script that he read in a porn magazine back when he was seventeen: "You are my slut-slave. I control everything you do. You will orgasm on command. I own you." And all that on the first date? C'mon. When I feel like what he is saying to me is the same thing he says to all his partners because he feels like "that's what a dom says," I definitely tune out. Contrary to what some people believe, there is no one way to be truly dominant. If you follow someone else's script, or use the same lines with every partner, or truly aren't sincere, that will probably be picked up on eventually.

Some tops have a tendency to get all hung up on technique, to worry that they haven't earned some mythical Top's Merit Badge. But topping has less to do with someone's level of experience and more about their creativity and level of engagement with what they're doing. If things are working right... if he's connected and intuitive and empathetic, I can be dropped to my knees by a look... and by a person who may have not the slightest idea of how to properly wield a flogger or what a singletail is. The greatest singletail expert in the world can be the most excruciatingly boring top if he's lacking in empathy. But most of my bottom friends tell me that the rawest newbie can grab their hair at just the right moment and turn their knees to jello with a kiss against a wall on Valencia Street.

There is an interesting conundrum that can come up with new tops. They need to learn somewhere. Unfortunately, some of them get caught up in the fact that they are dominant and don't want to be told anything. It can be very threatening to their egos. Classes are a great way for tops to get themselves educated. It's not as threatening and the BDSM organizations usually have pretty frequent classes taught by experienced people. There is also a wide variety of wonderful books on BDSM.

Tops can also go to pro-dommes for private instruction. Many tops will try bottoming as it gives them a perspective on what the other side feels like. Many good tops have bottomed at least once. It's hard to know what you're dishing out feels like if you've

> **KINKY GIRL TIP**
>
> *9 1/2 Weeks* was a sexy movie but food doesn't always have a place in play. I've watched someone try to get raspberry sauce off a deerskin flogger and it wasn't pretty.
>
> **KINKY GIRL TIP**

never been on the receiving end and it can be an *extremely* effective learning tool. Some tops will find a more experienced top to act as a mentor.

A top can also learn with a more experienced bottom but it can be tricky to provide instruction while maintaining the d/s power balance. The bottom has to be respectful of the top's ego and the top has to be not easily threatened. There's nothing quite like "hands-on" experience. As a bottom, I have occasionally stumbled over this problem with new tops. When I very respectfully suggested to one guy that his flogger strikes were a little high, he told me that I wasn't a "real submissive." (I then, not nearly so respectfully, informed him that "real submissives" have kidneys too and mine didn't appreciate being walloped.)

It seems to be easier for new submissives to learn. Many tops are more than pleased to act as mentors. I was lucky enough to happen upon a wonderful man who "showed me the ropes," so to speak, and taught me the safe, sane and consensual side of BDSM. He didn't have a lot of his own agenda wrapped up in it and was very patient and generous. Not everyone is so lucky.

ear Maddie,

Well, what's a girl to do... when she finds out she isn't always necessarily quite as much of a girl as she thought she was?

Yeah, yeah, it's another one of *those* stories. And it began like a lot of the rest of them: I had this guy tied up...

You know him, I think – Will, that sort of noisy little curly-haired guy who's always flirting with all the women at the munches. Come to think of it, all the men, too. You know we've played a couple of times – he's really a lot of fun, although it's always best to wear earplugs because he's not exactly the strong silent type –

"he turned his face and said, 'please, sir, will you call me bitch?'"

but I hardly need to tell you that, or anybody else who's played at any party in the San Francisco Bay Area (or probably Fresno either).

So we're at this party Friday night. Like I was saying, I had this guy tied up – to a St. Andrew's cross, as it happens. He was looking very sweet, with his back all red and blotchy from where I've been flogging it, and kind of panting after letting out a volley of squeals, and come to think of it I was breathing kind of hard myself and thinking about whether I could enter a flogging into my aerobics log.

I came up behind him for a big hug, pressing my sweaty tits against his hot steamy back as he winced and then sighed in contentment. And then, as I started to release him, he turned his head and said in a teeny little voice, "Please, Sir, will you call me 'bitch'?"

Oh my God, Maddie, I thought I was going to come and pass out and die, all at once, right there on the floor. I didn't even hesitate – I grabbed him again and began to hump his butt from behind, just as though I had a real honest-to-god cock. And right now as I write about it, I'm blushing, but at the time I wasn't; it felt as natural as could be: "That's right, bitch, show me how much you want it," I growled in his ear. "Move that pretty little ass of yours. Take every inch, you cunt…"

> **KINKY GIRL TIP**
>
> Some kinky girls aren't girly girls. If butch is your look and you want your breasts out of the way (or if you're playing with gender for fun), look in an out of the way place – a lingerie catalog. A "control thong" with the crotch piece cut off makes a good breast binder for small to midsize breasts.
>
> **KINKY GIRL TIP**

And he began to push back against me while I was humping him, and there we were, honest to god fucking, and all we needed was the genitals and we didn't really even need those. "Sir, oh sir, thank you sir…" was coming from somewhere out in the distance, and I heard sounds coming out of my throat that I didn't know my voice knew how to make, including something that sounded an awful lot like coming, except in a baritone. And somehow my face and belly flushed with blood, too – odd, that – and my knees went so weak that I almost fell down and had to grab onto Will and the cross for support.

So it looks like your girlfriend may be your boyfriend too – who knew? Will & I are going shopping together to-night – he's going to help me pick out my first dick and harness. I think I may go shopping for a nice pinstriped suit and tie sometime too. What do you think about the name "Sam"? I've always kind of liked it...

Love,

?

♥

Suki's about to discover something. Strapons are *cool*. Yep, you heard me correctly. Strapons are cool. The first time you gird your loins with one of those puppies you look at yourself in the mir-ror a *lot*. Once you're done with that, you wander around looking for things to stick it in. You become a teenage boy. Huh, well, maybe I'm universalizing my own experience. Seriously though, I think they rock. (If you think you might think so too, do a little reading up before you try one. Go slow, start small, and buy some good thick gooey water-based lube be-fore you hurt someone in the wrong way with that thing.)

Now, I'm not going to get all ex-Women's Studies Major on you, but playing with gender is fascinat-

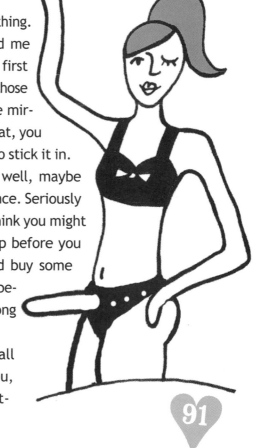

ing. Look at all the constructs our society builds on gender. Look at the power exchange that is frequently inherent in those constructs. Now fuck around with them. How fun is that?! We hear a lot about men playing with gender – transvestites, etc. Lesser known is the fact that many women, straight or not, enjoy playing with it as well. One girl I know gets kind of a thrill out of being called "Daddy." I know another woman, who's actually pretty vanilla *and* straight, who enjoys packing (wearing a strapon under her clothes) just because it makes her feel empowered. She doesn't *use* it, just wears it. In some lesbian relationships, the bottom is the "boi."

If you are playing with power dynamics, male versus female, the archetype of the strong male and more helpless female, try reversing that and put the top female in the male role, addressed with masculine terms and things can certainly heat up fast. Throw in some penetration and damn, it's taboo as hell but it can also send you over the moon. *You* get to be the penetrator, the fucker instead of the fuckee.

Some people also really enjoy having an alternate persona for play. It may be a little girl with pigtails but it may be the butchest construction worker you've ever seen.

Keep in mind, this is a powerful game you're playing and there may be repercussions. Take it slow and check in with your partner a *lot*. Some people may dream about being taken down by a hot woman with a cock but the reality of it can be overwhelming. Ladies, don't let your nine-inch dick lead you around by the nose.

Are you still a girl if you dream about wearing a cock? Does it make you wet to be called "Sir" or "Master?" Are you still straight if you want to get a blowjob? Sure, why not? Hey, I'm a girly-girl. I wear perfume, get pedicures *and* I have a strapon. But mine's pretty. It has silver glitter in it.

*M*addie and Carl are at a play party. They're not playing but are hanging out in the social area and idly chatting with a man who calls himself "Master Wolf." Rather, Carl is chatting with him and Maddie has tuned out. She's watching a wax play scene going on across the room and wondering to herself how you get wax out of your pubic hair. Suddenly her attention is caught by the conversation next to her.

"Coming on command?" Master Wolf says, "Sure. Watch this."

He whistles sharply

he growls into her ear, "come for me... now!"

and his submissive, Carrie, snaps to attention on the couch where she is sitting. She watches him attentively. He begins to count backwards from seven.

"Seven... six."

Carrie's head falls back and she begins to moan.

"Five... four..."

Her body begins to twist, her hands clench and she starts to breathe in little pants.

"Three... two..."

Her back arches and her nails claw at the fabric of the couch.

"ONE!"

Carrie's whole body convulses, her hips snap and she cries out apparently in throes of orgasm.

Maddie looks on in disbelief. Yeah, right... she is *so* faking that. No way in hell was that an actual orgasm. Maddie turns to Carl, expecting to see skepticism, but his mouth is hanging open and when he looks at her, she can see a gleam in his eye that bodes ill.

Later that night, Carl tries to hypnotize her, or something. "You will come for me when I command it. You will orgasm when I tell you to," he chants in a low soothing voice. Maddie looks at him doubtfully. "Um, OK," she answers, "I'll try." She goes into the bathroom to wash her face. As she is brushing her teeth, he comes up behind her and growls into her ear, "Come for me, girl. Come for me *now*!"

Maddie can't help it. Instead of orgasming she starts to giggle hysterically. She chokes on toothpaste and it spews all over the mirror. Carl looks furious. She tries to collect herself, to apologize with toothpaste dribbling down her chin, "I'm sorry...I'll try again..." It's no good, she starts laughing again and he stomps off to the bedroom.

Sometimes your top will ask you to do something that you just can't do, no matter how hard you try or how much you want to please him. One of my personal pet peeves is orgasming on command. I just can't do it and everyone seems to want it.

My orgasms take a little work and even then, they aren't guaranteed. They certainly don't fall out of the clear blue sky. I've seen people do it, or at least appear to do it (I always have my doubts), but it certainly has never happened to me.

For a long time, I was so eager to please, I just faked it. It's really no trouble at all, a little moaning, a little panting, work those Kegel muscles like a trouper and Ta-da!

> ## KINKY GIRL TIP
>
> So you dream of a hot pirate (think Johnny Depp in Pirates of the Caribbean - maybe a touch less fey) ripping the bodice from your heaving breasts? Or slicing neatly through your lace panties with a gleaming blade? Very hot, just make sure you're not wearing La Perla. I get distinctly testy when someone tries to rip off my pricey underwear. A friend who loves having her clothes ripped off stocks up on disposable clothes at Goodwill. Remember, if it's going to be shredded, bring something to wear home!
>
> ## KINKY GIRL TIP

I'm coming on command. Unfortunately, that can snowball on you. If they think they can make you come on command, they start pressing that button again and again and *again* and you can forget about them trying to get you off any other way. So as a punishment for being deceptive, you never get to actually come and are stuck in fake orgasm hell forever. It's a lose-lose situation.

If you can't do something, even if you don't have anything inherently *against* doing it, don't just fake it to please your partner. It'll catch up with you eventually and you'll certainly have more fun if you're both being realistic in your expectations.

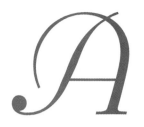

hhhh, negotiating. This can be a tough thing to learn. You're going to have to talk about all those things that good girls don't talk about. You're going to have to be clear about what you do and don't want even if you *really* want to be submissive and please your partner. One thing I would recommend, if your local BDSM organization has a class on negotiating, get your cute little butt in there ASAP. If they don't, you might want to try doing a little roleplay with some kinky friends before you try doing it for real so you don't end up all red-faced and stammering with no

3: how to negotiate a scene

bloody idea what you're doing.

First rule of negotiating. Don't wait until he's got you all tied up and is smacking the crop against his hand in anticipation. Negotiating should be done *before* you start playing, before the lust is turning your brain to mush. You want to be as clear-headed as possible and not in that delicious submissive head space. You need all your wits around you.

Come prepared. Think about your limits and don't let anyone persuade you to change them if you are not comfortable with that. These limits are *yours* and you do not need to explain or justify them to anyone. Hard limits are things you absolutely do not want to do and soft limits are things that scare you but you may want to try them eventually under the right circumstances. For a first scene with someone, it might be a good idea to start slow and not play with soft limits immediately. There are a lot of checklists out there – some of the books in the Resource Guide include good ones. These can be a great jumping off point for negotiating. They'll help you in case you forget to mention something. It will all be there in black and white while your face is turning red.

Yeah, there may be some amount of squirming involved in this process, it will become easier the more you do it, I promise. Women especially are taught to not be very explicit about their sexuality and desires in this society. Verbalizing all this stuff for the first time can be really hard. That's tough but you need to get over it. If you can't negotiate effectively, you can't take care of yourself and play within the boundaries of safety, sanity, and consensuality. You are ultimately in control of what happens to you no matter who has who tied up. Interestingly, you may find that learning how to do this may help you become a more effective negotiator in some of the vanilla areas of your life.

Remember that just because you are playing with someone does not mean you will fuck them. Your play actually does not have to be very sexual at all. Plenty of people go out and get a good flogging the way they would get a good massage. For other people it's fore-play. You are in control of the amount of sexual contact before, during, and after play.

Mention relevant medical issues or physical limitations during negotiations. Don't wait until you're hogtied to in-form your top about your trick knee, Whoops, there it goes!

Stick with your negotiations. Don't renegotiate in the middle of a scene to try something you had previously considered a limit. Endorphins do funny things to people, tops and bottoms, and good judgment frequently can fly out the window. If something seems like a great idea but wasn't part of your negotiating, store it away for a fu-ture negotiation, don't try to renegotiate on the fly with a bottom who is drooling in endorphin bliss. I've been so high on endorphins during a scene that I probably would have let someone cut off my ear if they felt like it. Fortu-nately, I had protected myself ahead of time and still have both my ears. Having said that, can you renegotiate out of something which you had said you wanted when you were sitting in that brightly-lit coffeeshop? This may seem hypocritical, but yes, you absolutely can. You may have thought you were ready for something but find out you really aren't, bad memories might get triggered, or you may simply just not be in the mood. When it comes to *not* doing previously-agreed-upon activities, you get to change your fickle little mind any time you please and a good partner will deal with it.

That brings us to safewords. Safewords are put in place in case something goes wrong in a scene. When

99

they are called, everything should come to a full screeching halt, toys should get dropped, bonds should be undone. They can be a word that would never come up in a regular scene. I had one top who used "asparagus" as a safeword. "No," "stop" and "ouch" are not generally good choices – many people like to use them and have the top keep on going; it's part of what makes the scene hot. On the other hand, if you like your "no" to mean "no," that's fine too, as long as you and your top both agree to that.

Safewords should be very very easy to remember. Many people use "safeword" as a safeword, and a lot of parties have "safeword" as a generic safeword that means "I need help from whoever hears me say this."

I'm a big fan of the "yellow" and "red" system. It gives you an option. "Yellow" can mean "slow down and check in." I use it if I'm not altogether comfortable and need to tell the top something but the scene doesn't necessarily have to end. It's also a great chance to mention something I might have forgotten during my negotiation but just remembered. Oops, sorry, nobody's perfect and I forgot to tell you if you bind my arms above my head for too long I will get dizzy and might just throw up all over that pretty new deerskin flogger. "Red" is the hard safeword and means it's time for that screeching halt mentioned above.

But what if you're gagged and can't say your safeword? Set up a silent safeword, a gesture of some sort. I have seen tops give the submissive a ball to hold and if they drop it they're calling safeword. I've also seen tops give the bottom a bell to ring.

Remember that anyone can call a safeword, top or bottom, for any reason. As a submissive, it used to be tough for me to call safeword because I felt like I was failing my top. I eventually realized that I was failing them more if I didn't safeword when I should have. Tops (brace yourself) are not infallible and they need to be able to trust their bottoms. I have a friend who can't safeword at all and she has to tell anyone who plays with her up front. Some people will not play with her because they do not want that responsibility.

If you're topping it's a good idea to check in with your bottom pretty frequently. This is especially true if you don't know them well and don't know how to read their reactions. Take a break in that crazy hot flogging and ask how they're doing, make sure they're still with you, ask them if they remember their safeword. Bottoms react differently during scenes. Some howl and fight and moan and cry and they're happy as a pig in shit. When I am processing heavy pain I sometimes get very still and quiet but I am just fine and having a great time. As you learn to read your bottom, you may have to check in less frequently. I love those moments when a top stops for a second, presses his body up against me, strokes my hair and whispers in my ear and... well... you know... check-ins can be fun.

If you're playing in public, or not at home, negotiate how you're going to get home. I've tried to drive after playing heavily and I might as well have had six shots of tequila and gotten behind the wheel. I almost hit a pedestrian and then got terribly lost on a route I knew very well and started heading down a freeway in the absolute wrong direction in the middle of the night. My brain was quite definitely addled and I shouldn't have been in control of any sort of vehicle. Are you going to spend the night with them at their place? Will they drive you home? Will you plant your bruised behind in a cab? Will you flaunt your fetishwear on the subway? Figure it out in advance. Maybe you're hardcore and could safely operate a Lear Jet after playing. I found out the hard way that I'm not. Good thing that pedestrian was alert.

Aftercare is something you may also want to include in your negotiations. This part frequently gets forgotten. It can take some time to come down from a scene, both for the top and the bottom. Some repercussions may not fully develop until the next day, or a few days later. You may be someone who just needs twenty minutes of cuddling after a scene. It's usually not a good idea to try to talk about real-world stuff, or to discuss the scene and how it went, too soon afterwards – just drift together and enjoy the afterglow. I won't do a heavy scene with someone unless I know that we can spend the night together.

As a top, checking in with your bottom the next day by phone is a really good idea. You have shared an experience and that experience doesn't fully end when the key unlocks the cuffs. That's part of the beauty of it.

*M*addie is pretty heavy. She doesn't think of herself as obese but she is probably within a stone's throw. She prefers "Rubenesque."

Before she starts going to play parties and munches, she fears that all the women will look like Barbie dolls in fetishwear – that's what she's seen in the movies. The reality is much much different. All sorts of bodies, all over the place. Not only that but all sorts of people finding those bodies sexy! Even better, there are plenty of people who find her body sexy and tell her so.

Not every reaction is

*he tells her that he **misses** those ample **hips**...*

positive, of course. She goes on one date through a personal ad website. She has described herself as "voluptuous" and "curvy" in her ad and she thinks that is pretty accurate. She gets dressed up in a pretty new sundress that shows off her ample cleavage. When the guy arrives, he looks her up and down, doesn't even bother concealing the disappointment in his eyes, and barely speaks to her all through lunch, obviously ready to go out and look for the thinner model. That hurts. That hurts a lot. But Maddie recovers. She certainly is not hurting for people to play with.

Maddie does end up losing some weight. She starts going to the gym, eating differently. Not because of one blind date gone wrong, but for her own health reasons. She wants to be able to ride a bike, to ski. The reactions from people in the BDSM community vary.

Some people start noticing her who had never noticed her when she was heavier. Some eyes that looked right through her as if she was invisible before, light on her appreciatively now. While she likes the attention, she never quite trusts these people.

> **KINKY GIRL TIP**
>
> Eating out of a doggie bowl is difficult if you are choking on your own hair. Tie back those lovely locks, you naughty puppy!
>
> **KINKY GIRL TIP**

One guy she used to play with tells her she looks great. She gets a phone call from him later that night. "You know how I told you how great you look?" he asks, "I just wanted to let you know that I always thought you were beautiful." She is absurdly touched that he called to tell her this.

Another friend gives her a hug and then openly bemoans the shrinking of her once luscious breasts. She actually likes that. He tells her that he misses those ample hips, that bottom that begged to be smacked. The part of her who is still that heavier girl adores him for it. She'll never be skinny, she'll always be a big girl, she knows that. She also comes to realize that there will be people who want her no matter what her weight.

♥

Just like in the vanilla world, there will always be people who want that perfect prototype. You know the one: young, high perfect tits that defy gravity, impossible measurements. Ironically, the guys seeking that model are often far from ideal themselves, with guts hanging out over their too-tight leather pants. Don't worry about it, let them look.

The truth of the matter is that there are people out there who will find you sexy if you find yourself sexy. They'll lust after you with your extra padding, graying hair, stretch marks and cellulite. They'll know that an ample bottom just makes a better target. If you're thin, there will also be people who want to devour you.

And whatever your body type, there will be people for whom you're a fetish object – for whom your big (or small) breasts, or bottom, or feet, or ears, or hair, or whatever, are going to seem more important than *you*. Or maybe it'll be your height, or your age, or your race that's attracting them, and you may feel sort of secondary to whatever their kink may be. You'll have to decide for yourself how you feel about that – it can be fun and playful, or really hurtful. One friend of mine, who is chunkier than social norms but far from obese, tells about dating a guy whose preference was for really big women, and having decidedly mixed emotions: on one hand, she says, she felt sort of bummed that he found her body less than attractive, but on the other hand it was an amazing feeling to go out with someone who thought she was too skinny!

The important thing is that you stay healthy and enjoy your own body. If you know you're hot, not enough to be an arrogant bitch about it, but enough to be comfortable and self-assured in your own skin, you will be the embodiment of sexy for a lot of people.

If someone doesn't want to play with you because you're too fat, thin, old, short, whatever, let them go. They're entitled to their preferences. You will have much more pleasurable experiences with people that delight in you just as you are.

he man appears to be in the the throes of a monumental orgasm in the middle of his living room floor. He is moaning and literally writing on the olive green carpet. Maddie feels like she shouldn't be watching, it seems terribly rude to observe what should be a very private moment, but she also can't look away. It is like watching a car crash. A very embarrassing car crash.

She sits on the overstuffed couch and gnaws a thumbnail nervously and tries to figure out how she has gotten there. It is not a situation she has ever imagined herself in. Maybe if

*she wasn't **sure** whether to watch him **writhing** or to look the **other** way...*

she can figure out how she got there, she can figure out how to get herself out. She wishes he would be a little quieter. She watches the rug bunching up under his body. From the other side of the room, his small gray cat looks on dispassionately. Maddie wonders how often the cat has seen this particular demonstration.

... She met him at a munch in Berkeley. He seemed reasonably intelligent, attractive, and polite. She liked the way his eyes looked when he smiled at her. He asked her to dinner and she accepted.

They went for Indian food and had a perfectly pleasant time. She did experience a brief moment of discomfort when he tried (unsuccessfully) to demonstrate Tuvan throat singing at the dinner table. There was a lull in the noise level at the restaurant and some other diners turned to look when he made an odd squawking sound. Maddie blushed but he didn't notice.

They negotiated a playdate for the following week as he kissed her goodbye against her old car. She looked forward to the date, sort of. He seemed a little "crunchy" or "New Age" but she would remain open-minded. The kiss had been good, after all, and he had pressed against her hard.

The next week she went up to his house, nestled into the Berkeley hills. He let her in and didn't grab her immediately but wanted to talk. He had spoken about tantra when they had dinner and he asked if she would like to try some "exercises." Sure, why not throw a little education in with her sex?

He had her stand at one end of the room and then he walked toward her until she raised her hands and said "no." Then he wanted to know exactly what she felt at the moment he crossed some invisible boundary.

She couldn't tell him the truth: she feels dumb doing exercises like this and also that he had such a strange look in his eyes when he crossed toward her that she suddenly couldn't bear the thought of his hands on her. She stammered something about feeling him enter her space and felt foolish but he appeared satisfied with her answer.

Then he wanted to show her the "tantric undulation." It didn't sound like this was going anywhere good but she agreed and sat on the couch where he indicated. He lay down on the floor and started by describing his breathing. Then he started rotating his pelvis. She picked at a hangnail. Gradually his whole body started to undulate as she stared. He began moaning and his eyes rolled up in his head. There she was, watching the car wreck...

She remembers a fish her father had caught writhing in a bucket on the floor of his boat. Her father had eventually put the fish out of its misery by smacking it on the head with an old bat. The fish flopped a couple more times and then lay still, its eyes glazing over. This man also looks like he is drowning in air. She suspects smacking him on the head with a bat is not a valid option although if he isn't careful, he's going to hit his head on the coffee table. She almost giggles but manages to keep a straight face. He seems to come to sort of

KINKY GIRL TIP

Blindfolds can wreak havoc on the most artfully applied makeup. If you're as vain and silly as I am and don't want to look like a raccoon, go with waterproof. Along those lines, hoods ruin hairdos. Bring a brush. Or you can borrow the one that was just used to paddle your bottom.

KINKY GIRL TIP

a peak and then subsides at her feet. Has he come? The cat, possibly sensing that the show is over, gets up and stretches one leg and then another and then strolls out of the room. Maddie envies it and thinks longingly of her car which is parked outside.

As he gets up and comes toward her, Maddie's brain starts to scramble frantically for a way to get out of there with some measure of grace. She couldn't possibly feel less submissive to this man at this point. He fumbles with her blouse and she cringes and starts to stammer his own words back at him. Words like "boundaries" and "feeling safe enough to say no." He actually thanks her for being so clear with her boundaries while looking a little disappointed. Then he wants to hold her while they both "decompress." She lies with him stiffly, afraid that any movement would be seen as a sign of encouragement. She stays only as long as seems polite. When he starts to nuzzle her neck and she feels his breathing change, she disengages herself and heads for the door. She escapes while he is still looking confused.

There will be activities, kinks and fetishes that you had no idea existed. People you play with will suddenly come up with stuff you had no clue they were into. Sometimes it will jibe well with your own kink if you leave yourself open to it. Who knew Daddy/little girl play could be so much fun? Sometimes you may find yourself being accommodating to please a lover. Tying them upside down and tickling them with an ostrich feather can be mildly entertaining, and it makes them *so* happy. Sometimes it may just *not* be what you're into and completely turn you off.

I started playing with one guy, not realizing he had any gender dysphoria issues. One day we were preparing to attend a fetishwear event and he wanted to go in drag. I didn't think he would make a particularly pretty woman but I wasn't upset. When he spent the entire day depilating his rather hirsute body, I became more perturbed. When he asked me to shave his back, I was outright dismayed. Apparently I was more squeamish than I had realized. The relationship was short-lived and she is now a pre-op transsexual. When it comes right down to it, I would prefer a male top without gender dysphoria issues. Other people prefer transgendered partners.

One top loved to get his cock sucked, every morning, for an *hour*. He would set the alarm early and there would be a command performance to start his day. I loved to please him and would groggily comply. Fortunately we split up (for other reasons) before the onset of TMJ.

A friend's lover never had penis/vagina intercourse, only anal.

Some of these accommodations seem relatively minor in the face of larger differences. What if you're a bottom and fall in love with another bottom? Everything else is right but the sexual dynamic of your relationship doesn't click. Either you both learn to switch, embrace polyamory at least to some extent, or face a partnership of denial and frustration.

Another person may have been fascinated by the tantra demonstration. It could have been a doorway into a whole other world of sexuality. Someone else might have indulged this man's predilection. It just didn't work for Maddie. Watching that man writhe on the floor had the effect of a bucket of cold water on her libido. Maybe it was her sexually conservative New England upbringing poking its prudish head out of her psyche. Whatever it was, she was turned *off* by that particular form of sexual expression. She wants to please her partners but there are places she doesn't want to go. No tantric undulation, apparently.

111

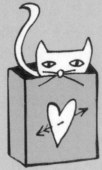

KINKY GIRL TIP

Pets and your kink. Kitties love floggers and puppies adore leather. Keep them out of the toybag and away from your scene. I once had a cat take a playful swipe at a chain which happened to be attached to clamps which happened to be attached to my nipples. The top thought it was funny, I wasn't so amused.

KINKY GIRL TIP

The world of kink encompasses such a broad range of sexuality, the chances of finding one person who is tailor-made to your kink can seem impossible – and may well be. As in most relationships, kinky or vanilla, some compromises usually have to be made. You need to decide how much you can or should adjust. If your partner wants a 24/7 relationship and you don't want that sort of dynamic, maybe playing with it on weekends would work for both of you. Figure out how much you can compromise and still end up happy and satisfied.

ear Maddie,

Well, I guess maybe the old chestnut about old dogs and new tricks isn't true – or else I'm not that old a dog yet. Who knew?

So it all began Saturday night. I was at the play party with Larry – you were there too, but you looked much too busy to be paying attention to what I was up to, lucky girl – and his old playpartner Shawna was there. Don't know if you remember her – looks like a cross between Venus of Willendorf and the Appalachian Range, just six big broad feet of hips and breasts and thighs and tummy and hair, and *so* smart and funny.

> *"big soft breasts, and a pussy... well, i didn't dare think about that just yet..."*

Anyway, turns out it was her birthday. And I think she must have had the idea that Larry was going to play with her, but he, being your typical tungsten-skulled testosterone case, hadn't gotten the message, or something – anyway, he was off drooling over the latest Sweet Young Thing and hardly even knew Shawna was there. So she and I were chatting, but she knew I didn't play with girls, and I could tell by the way her eyes kept drifting away over my shoulder that a chat with me wasn't really high up on her list of ways she wanted to while away the first night of her 34th year, you know?

113

So we drifted on to other things. But an hour later, I saw her with her coat on and her toybag in her hand, about to open the door and go, with the saddest slump to her shoulders you ever saw in your life, and Maddie, hetero-girl or no, I just couldn't let that happen.

"Shawna!" I called. "You're not *leaving!* Not without your birthday scene!"

She turned around, her face brightening... and the next thing you knew, there we were: her stripped naked, with her hands tied over her head, her feet tied at either end of a three-foot spreader bar, and me with the contents of my bag spread around like presents under a very large pink tree on Christmas morning. And somewhere down in the middle of my feelings of panic, I had to be honest with myself: this woman was *hot*. Big soft breasts with huge pink nipples, a belly to bury yourself in, thighs like confectionery... and a pussy... well, I didn't really even dare think about that just yet... it was all too confusing. But one thing, at least, I knew what to do with: I stretched upward and planted a big, gentle, wet kiss on the softest, deepest lips I'd ever kissed in my life. I had to stretch to reach all the way around her big warm body, but oh, it was worth it.

OK, Suki: you've got her, now what the hell are you going to do with her? I looked down at the toys at my feet. There lay a bag of clothespins I'd bought recently and hadn't even had a chance to open yet – far too many clothespins for most bottoms, but Shawna had so much real estate... was it possible? Well, I could at least try a few and see how it went...

I started with the big pillowy breasts. A few around the outside, in the places that on my breasts would be relatively easy to tolerate. (Would someone else's breasts have the same feelings in the same places as mine? How can you know?) She sighed, swayed, started to move her hips a bit. More clothespins, then – she moistened her lips and I saw her labia part a bit. Hey, I think I'm getting the hang of this.

Shawna was responsive, masochistic, easy to read – your basic joy. Working in a measured pace, stopping occasionally for a kiss or caress, it took me maybe fifteen or twenty minutes to place the entire package of fifty clothespins all over the front of her big soft body – breasts, belly, thighs, even a few on that tantalizing pussy (I could hardly believe I was touching it). By then, I was breathing almost as hard as she was – and clothespins are no physical work

KINKY GIRL TIP

Fetishwear ain't designed to be comfy for the most part; it's designed to look hot. You may find that you would rather chew off your left foot than be strapped back into that gorgeous corset or wriggle back into that latex after a hot scene. If you're weak in the knees, six-inch stilettos are hazardous as hell. Take it from someone who has fallen on her sore ass more than once. Toss a teeshirt and some flats into that toybag!

KINKY GIRL TIP

at all; my breathing was pure arousal. I stood back to look at my handiwork – the ivory of her skin darkening to peach around each pin, the flush of turn-on on her chest, neck and face, the gleam of moisture between her labia.

I was overwhelmed with affection and lust – feelings I'd rarely felt for a man, and never, of course, for a woman – and then I know just what to do. What do you do with a feeling like that, but a great, big, loving, bearhug?

I stepped up to her and took her in my arms. I hugged her tightly to me – grinding every single clothespin agonizingly into her flesh. She let out a wailing moan of pleasure and pain that made me clutch her to me even closer, tightening my fingertips into her back, pushing my knee between her legs, never wanting to let her go. A sudden moisture on my leg – I'd always thought that the expression "dripping pussy" was a pornographer's exaggeration, but I learned differently in that moment (when I cleaned up after the scene, I found an actual puddle on the ground).

I never asked her if she came at that moment – I've always hated being nagged about whether or not I've come – but I think she probably did. Happy birthday, Shawna.

Then, of course, the exquisite joy of removing all the clothespins, one by one, as I stroked her face and consoled her during her cries of pain.

"Old dog," indeed. Shawna and I have a date for next Saturday night. How have I missed out on half the human race for all these years??!!

Your newly awakened friend,

Suki

116

♥

Ah, the joys of discovery! Suki is blessed with an open mind and a great imagination. These led her to new realms of her own sexuality which she had not previously explored.

Maybe you've never played with women before, maybe it's something you have no desire to do. But maybe there's a flicker of interest. Hell, maybe you've been secretly getting yourself off to the idea for years.

The BDSM scene is pretty accepting of many different forms of sexuality – it can be a great place to experiment. It was Suki's first time playing with a woman and she was sort of stymied. She followed her instincts and went with what was comfortable for her and seemed to come naturally. Any scene that results in a puddle on the floor... well... need I say more?

Don't agonize over labels. Are you bisexual if you just play with women in public? Do you only fuck girls if there's a guy involved? Do you only fuck guys if there's a girl around? Are you straight if you love being cuddled into pillowy breasts? Can you

117

really be a dyke if you like being spanked by a guy? Who cares if everyone's consenting and everyone's turned on? Think outside *the* box when using *your* box and the possibilities are almost endless.

*G*eoff is a "newbie." He has just discovered BDSM, just gone to his first munch, wants more of what he is beginning to taste and wants it immediately.

He is so eager to go to the club, it makes Maddie a little nervous. She would rather go to a movie, go to dinner a few times. She wants to get to know him a little better, maybe play a few times. Ease him into things.

She can sympathize. She remembers the sense of urgency and impatience when she discovered this world existed. He wants to see it all right *now*. He wants her to show it to him.

She rounds up Larry and Suki, who go to that club frequently. With reinforcements

geoff is fascinated with the club, but it seems like a morbid fascination...

she feels a little less pressured. Geoff is so excited, it radiates off him in waves. To Maddie, it has a whiff of desperation. Nothing can possibly live up to his expectations.

She wears one of Suki's corsets because she doesn't have time to go home and get her own clothes. Suki is shaped differently and Maddie feels self-conscious about how her hips look under the brocade. Suki is also bustier than she is: she has to keep pulling her breasts up into the cups. Geoff wants to feel her waist through the stiff fabric. He tells her it makes him hard and she flushes with pleasure and embarrassment.

119

They all go to the club together. She has only been a couple of times before. There are a lot of voyeurs, men wandering around with towels wrapped around their waists. Even in the dim and lurid lighting, she can see the discomfort writhing behind some of their eyes. Others appear perfectly in their element. They stare openly and frankly at her. It is almost as if she has given over her body to them just by showing up. She takes Geoff's hand, feeling less and less like the authority.

One man masturbates constantly. She has seen him there before, eternally rubbing himself, so terribly proud of his own cock. She wonders what he does by day. Is he sore while he is at work? Does he ever tire of the feeling of his own cock in his hand? He sees her watching him and turns towards her as if offering himself for inspection. She doesn't meet his eyes.

Geoff is fascinated with the entire place. She watches him looking at everything and answers his questions to the best of her ability. It seems like a morbid fascination rather than open-minded acceptance. She starts to feel vaguely worried again. It isn't her favorite club but it doesn't cause her any particular dismay. She wonders about his kink, why is he here exactly. There seems to be some judgment in his tone.

Finally she has to leave: she has to get up early the following day. Geoff wants to stay. Larry and Suki are going to play and he wants to watch. He kisses her goodbye and she feels him hard against her and wants to stay.

After she gets home and climbs into bed, the phone rings. It is one a.m. She answers it quickly, her stomach suddenly tight with worry. It has to be an emergency for someone to call so late.

It is Geoff, apologetic but very upset. A story spills out of him, somewhat fragmented, but coherent enough that she is able to put together a picture of what has happened. Larry and Suki played. It was very intense, involving a lot of physical pain and some heavy humiliation. Geoff watched, not really understanding that it was all consensual and prenegotiated. To him, it looked like abuse. Both Larry and Suki appeared to him to be psychotic. Nothing is as he had thought it would be and it upsets him. She listens and tries to explain, tries to help him understand, but he hangs up still distraught.

He speaks to her a few more times but the casual intimacy and affection are gone. He has become distant and withdrawn, sure there is something inherently wrong with anyone involved with that world. She protests half-heartedly. How can he judge her when she hadn't even been there? She gives up quickly because he doesn't seem worth the trouble and she doesn't like how quick he is to judge. Finally he calls to ask if she wants to go to coffee. She never calls him back.

Introducing people to the world of BDSM can be tricky. Frequently, the image they have in their heads, an image reinforced by the media, is pretty far from reality. Seeing other people play can be harrowing for the newcomer. Activities that are actually fully consensual can look brutal and abusive.

What they see and what they're feeling and maybe desiring is very taboo in our society. It's tougher for some people to get past that. Others seem to take to it like a fish to water. I've seen some people play for the first time, have a fantastic scene, and wake up the next morning racked with guilt and

121

remorse. I took to things fairly readily. I would however, on occasion, wonder if something was wrong with me. Usually, at the beginning, I was too turned on to care.

If the person you're introducing to BDSM is a close friend, a lover, someone you care about, be aware that their own self-doubts can sometimes manifest in judgments about *you*. This can be very difficult. If Maddie had been closer to Geoff, his condemnation could have been devastating to her.

In my experience, the best way to introduce a "newbie" to the scene is to do it gradually, rather than dumping them into the deep end of the pool. Try giving them a reading list. It may not be the hard core ass-whipping they were hoping for on the first date but it'll be good for them. There is a list of great books in the Resource Guide at the back of this book. Make yourself available for questions. Make sure they pick up on the "safe, sane and consensual" part. If they watch people play, it might be less shocking if they comprehend that what they're witnessing is done on the basis of informed consent.

Encourage them to go to munches and classes. It was a revelation to me how *normal* a lot of other kinky people are. They aren't a bunch of intimidating creatures walking around with needles stuck through them and permanently clad in latex (although a few of those exist – be careful around them, latex rips pretty easily and ripped latex makes them cranky).

It can be great for someone to have a more experienced mentor during this process of discovery. For the person doing the guiding, it can feel like a lot of responsibility. It also can be fun, you sort of rediscover things through their eyes. I know one woman who almost specializes in bringing new dominants into the scene. She seems to do a beautiful and graceful job of it. Maddie, on the other hand, felt like a failure in her role as mentor for Geoff.

*M*addie loves her mother – an amazing woman who really did her best to prepare Maddie for all sorts of situations. Maddie knows which fork to use at dinner, how to write a thank you note, all sorts of protocols for polite society. She has discovered, however, that there are many situations in the life that she is living that her mother did not prepare her for – granted, they are situations most mothers could never have dreamed of. Hell, they are usually situations that Maddie could not have dreamed of. But they keep on happening.

Maddie likes to think of

"oh my god, you've chopped it off!" she almost screamed...

herself as relatively unshockable, especially when it comes to sex and sexuality. Not that she's jaded, mind you – just, well – she's been part of the SM community for a while and lives in the San Francisco Bay Area. She has discovered she can still be shocked. It's sort of a good thing, she's not completely jaded. When she becomes totally unfazed by anything, she'll start to worry.

She doesn't usually top. It just doesn't have the same mouth-watering, knee-melting charge to it that she gets when she bottoms. There is something intoxicating about topping,

123

the power has its own rush to it, but it doesn't make her wet. She feels an almost scientific detachment when she tops. It brings her more into her head rather than driving her out of it.

Pete has convinced her to do some topping. He is an immensely appealing guy, sweet and engaging. He has had a bunch of different careers, all of them high-powered and fascinating. He is brilliant with a dry wit and delivers his jokes with a sharp sarcasm that she adores. He has many of the qualities that she is looking for. There are a few major drawbacks. He is married and has a kid. He also is a bottom. The marriage isn't an obstacle to their playing together. It is a polyamorous relationship with very few restrictions. Maddie has met his wife, who has a long-term lover who actually lives with them. All very civilized. Pete isn't relationship material for Maddie because she doesn't want to be a secondary partner.

His being a bottom is more of a problem. But he wants to play with her with a ferocity that is almost overwhelming. The attention is flattering and she thinks it is worth a shot. She doesn't have any other play partners at the moment and she is a little restless and a little horny. He writes her some emails with some of his fantasies and they sort of intimidate her in their extremity.

She enjoys playing with him. He hands over power so completely, surrenders to her so utterly that it is irresistible. He whimpers when she touches him and looks up at her with a soft vulnerability in his eyes, so open that it amazes her. Their play is sporadic. He comes over about once a month and guides her through the process of doing terrible things to him. He loves it. He even teaches her to fist him. Rather than being grossed out, the feel of him around her hand, so tight and warm, makes her feel like she has accomplished something. Then the sense of responsibility overwhelms her and she wants his body lying on top of her. Apparently her desire for control is finite.

Sometimes her own sadism frightens her. She hurts him and watches dispassionately as he moans and writhes, trying to process the pain as the welts come up on his inner thighs. He begs for mercy and she just watches with a slight smile. Even though it is what he wants, she occasionally finds herself overcome with remorse afterwards.

He is a man covered with evidence of his extreme desires. He has brands and tattoos covering his body, as well as multiple piercings. She lies in bed with him, running her fingers over the ridges in his skin and wonders what he had felt at the moment of infliction. Was he hard when the branding iron struck him? Some of his body modifications she doesn't particularly like. The brands look twisted and asymmetrical to her and feel jagged under her fingers. He likes it when she yanks on the heavy rings threaded through his flesh.

One day he walks through the door looking extraordinarily pleased with himself. He wants to show her his newest chastity device. He likes having his erections controlled and used to run a shackle through the piercing at the tip of his cock and around his balls so he couldn't get hard without it hurting. She is curious as to what new device he has come up with.

So he pulls out his penis. Or what appears to be left of his penis. The organ displayed is a mere fraction of what she remembers and has a bit of surgical tape across the tip. She stands there horrified. The man has amputated his penis. A voice screams inside her head "He's chopped it off! He's chopped it OFF!!" as she struggles to not show her emotions on her face. It feels like she was wearing a rigid brittle mask. It is not outside the realm of possibility for him to have it removed for his own unfathomable reasons. He has even had the flap of skin underneath his tongue snipped to make it longer. Why wouldn't he amputate his cock?

She doesn't want to hurt his feelings but she is truly shocked and has no idea what to say. What he wants to do with his body, even if he has Lorena Bobbitted himself, you shouldn't really criticize them should you? It's their choice and all that. Maddie keeps a poker-straight face and very politely says "What's this?" (It should be noted that this phrase works beautifully in all sorts of baffling situations.) Well, it turns out that he hasn't amputated it at all. Merely managed to invert the tip of it and tape it down so that erections become somewhere between painful and impossible. Interesting. Odd, but interesting. Certainly not as disturbing as the other option.

He wears this new device as they go out to dinner and Maddie never tells him she thought for a moment that he had taken his body modifications to a new level.

Sometimes you will have a partner whose fantasies are at a different level than yours. Sometimes they will mesh enough that you can make it work between you. Sometimes it's so far off that there seems to be no common ground. Pete's fantasies were kind of hard core for Maddie. He was into some stuff that she didn't want to touch,

> **KINKY GIRL TIP**
>
> White, powdery deodorant makes a mess on black clothing. Go for the clear gel versions.
>
> **KINKY GIRL TIP**

he would happily venture into areas where she didn't want to set foot.

But what do you do if you meet your soulmate and you're both bottoms, or both tops? Or he/she's married? Or (gasp) vanilla? Or monogamous when you want to be poly? What if the reality is not part of your fantasies?

Well, you can sometimes adjust your fantasy to fit with reality, but it's sometimes tougher to bend reality to fit your fantasy.

If you're both bottoms or tops, you can try stuff like flipping a coin to see who's on top that day, or week, or whatever. I know one couple where one partner topped for several years and then they decided to switch and now the other partner has been the top for the last few years. But maybe you have no desire to switch, not now, not ever. You're a bottom, goddammit, and a bottom you will stay. Well, you either need to accept the fact that you and your partner will not get your needs met completely or you will have to look for alternate ways to get those needs met. Some people with vanilla partners go to pro-dommes, or have kinky partners they play with, preferably with their partner's permission. If you're both bottoms or tops, you may want to work out some arrangement by which you can play with other people that fit your orientation.

If your partner is married and wants to stay married and you have a healthy polyamorous thing going where everyone's being honest and communicative then there may be no problem. If you're seeing a married person behind the spouse's back, well, I don't need to tell you that's sticky. Figure it out and find another soul mate.

I've seen a lot of people struggle with the poly/monogamous issue and I've struggled with it myself. It's tough, no two ways about it. If you're monogamous and fall in love with a poly person, or vice versa, you've got a lot of painful conversations ahead of you. You may decide that it's worth it and you can work it out or you may decide that this is not the match for you after all. Check the Resource Guide for help in finding books, therapists and so on.

*M*addie had tried to be bisexual in college. She had gone through a nasty breakup with a guy and she had an idea in her head that women would be nicer to each other. She started taking classes in the Women's Studies department. She decided everyone was born bisexual and socialized into their heterosexual roles. She stopped shaving her legs, although she couldn't quite bring herself to stop shaving her armpits. There was a group of lesbians who always ate in her dining hall and they were fascinating. They looked so... well... confident and strong. She studied them from afar. She tried hard to get a

suddenly her front teeth were shoved up against a pussy...

crush on one of them and half-convinced herself that it was working.

Later, she fooled around with other women a couple of times. It was fine, kissing a woman was not much different than kissing a man, maybe softer somehow. No facial hair. Nothing ever went very far because the erotic charge just wasn't as powerful as when she was with a guy and she had no desire to eat pussy, which she assumed was kind of a requirement. She ended up with some close dyke friends and watched them go through their own tribulations and figured out that relationships with women weren't any less difficult than heterosexual relationships. Everyone ends up in tears at some point no matter what gender you're fucking.

She wound up deciding that she was probably pretty straight and that wasn't really a problem for her. Until she got into the scene.

"So," he asks on their first date, "have you ever been with another woman?" She tells him that she had messed around with some girls in college and his eyes light up. She gets wary immediately. There seems to be a presumption (or so she believes) that if you're a submissive woman, you should automatically be bisexual and perfectly happy to fool around with any woman your dom decides to present you with.

> **KINKY GIRL TIP**
>
> Turn off your cell phones and pagers before you play. Nothing pisses your partner of more than a ringing cell phone, except you answering that ringing cell phone when they're about to have a great big orgasm.
>
> **KINKY GIRL TIP**

"I really don't think I'm bisexual," she says. "It just doesn't really do it for me."

"Uh-huh," he replies, with a faraway look in his eyes. "Did it disgust you?"

"No," she says slowly, because it hadn't. She remembers a light-hearted game of spin the bottle. "It was fun. It just never went anywhere. I'm pretty straight."

He looks at her speculatively but drops the subject.

A couple of months later, they go to a play party. They've played a few times and their chemistry is pretty good. His touch is strong and demanding and she finds herself wanting to please him. He strips her and attaches her to a leash. She kneels beside him while he chats with some people. She studies his toes and he pats her head absentmindedly. That makes her wet. Finally he feels like playing and he pulls her over his knee and spanks her hard. He talks to her softly as he fingers her. "Do you want to make me happy? Do you want to make me hard? Do you want to make me come?" She cries out yes yes YES and that *is* all she wants suddenly. His voice rumbles in her ear and she moans. Suddenly the world goes dark as he blindfolds her and he stands up... pulling on the leash. She follows him, stumbling a little, trying hard to be graceful and pliant.

He stops and tells her to kneel down. He's gone for a moment and she thinks she can hear him speaking to someone else. She cannot hear what is being said, the music is too loud. Suddenly he is behind her. His hand twists in the hair at the nape of her neck and pulls her head back. She gasps as her back arches. His voice is purring in her ear again. "Make me happy. Make me proud."

Then her face is pushed forward into a cunt. She freezes. She was completely unprepared for it. They hadn't negotiated this and she had thought their little conversation about her not being bisexual had been kind of clear. A woman moans above her and squeezes her thighs around Maddie's head. Maddie doesn't know what to do. She feels the wetness on her face and pulls back instinctively but can't get far. His hand is still on the back of her head. "Make me proud." She swims in confusion. After what seems like hours, she opens her mouth and tries a few experimental licks. She finds the woman's clitoris and the anonymous woman starts writhing and moaning louder. Maddie wants nothing so much as to be at home, alone, in her own bed in her fuzzy pajamas with her teddy bear and a good book. She tries to think about that, tries not to think about how her knees are starting to hurt on the cold cement floor. Tears start up in her eyes because she feels betrayed and hurt. She wants to stop but some part of her still doesn't want to disappoint him and she also doesn't want to hurt the feelings of who-ever this woman is. If someone were eating *her* out and started crying she would feel terrible. So she holds it all together and tries to get it over with. It's not as if it's repulsive, it's really not. It's just not where she wants to be.

Finally, after an eon, the woman's thighs squeeze harder for a moment and then release. Apparently she has come and now it's over. He pulls Maddie back. They both pet and stroke her for a moment. The blindfold is still on. After a few seconds, she is led away. She wants to wash her face. He stands in front of her and removes the blindfold. He looks utterly delighted with himself and she can see his erection. "That was so *hot,*" he murmurs, pulling her close. Maddie stiffens and pulls away. Suddenly pleasing him doesn't seem so important anymore. "I want to go home," she says. He takes her home and she doesn't ask him in. She washes her face immediately with very hot water. Then she finds the pack of cigarettes she keeps for emergencies. She smokes one on the balcony, blowing the smoke out into the rain. Then she goes inside, takes a shower, puts on her fuzzy PJ's and goes to bed alone.

There are a couple of lessons in this story. You need to be very very clear in your negotiations. Maddie thought that their conversation about her sexuality would just make it clear that she wasn't bi and that would be the end of it. She never bothered to spell it out as a hard limit because she just assumed that he would know. That was a mistake. Now, her partner was at fault as well. This is a hot-button scene to try without advance negotiation. If he had asked her in advance whether this was something she wanted to try, she would most likely made it pretty clear that it wasn't and she wouldn't have ended up in the middle of a very uncomfortable situation.

Now, she had the option of safewording in the middle of the scene. Someone later, hearing the story, asked her why she hadn't. Maddie started to cry at that point because it was the first time it had even

> **KINKY GIRL TIP**
>
> I love "pearl necklaces" as much as the next girl but not while I'm wearing a $200 satin corset.
>
> **KINKY GIRL TIP**

occurred to her. In her mind, safewords were only to be used in moments of life-threatening physical emergencies. The possibility hadn't even crossed her mind at the time. Safewords can be used at any time, not just when your physical health is threatened. If a scene is going bad for you in

133

any way, if something is coming up emotionally, slow things down and talk about it before continuing. In retrospect, Maddie should have "yellowed" and then told this guy that she wasn't up for this, thank you very much.

Many people in the BDSM scene, men and women alike, do often seem to be bisexual. There is a lot of acceptance for all sorts of sexual variance. But you don't *have* to be. If you want to experiment with it, that's great. If you don't, that's also great.

The same applies to polyamory. Your dom may want you to be OK with playing or sleeping with other people. He may want to play or sleep with other people himself. This may be just fine with you. You may be able to negotiate certain agreements that make it just fine with you. You may not. If you don't want to play or sleep with other people and expect the same from your partner, that's your choice. Always operate within your comfort levels. Polyamory may not be your thing. Maybe you've tried it and it didn't work for you, maybe you have no desire to go there. There's no rulebook that says you have to be polyamorous to be kinky. Operate within your comfort levels and don't allow anyone, no matter how hot or persuasive, to talk you into doing things you don't want to. Chances are, you'll end up resenting that person and yourself, for getting you into a situation you didn't want to be in. It is best to be clear with this stuff up front. If someone presents himself as polyamorous and you know you're not, tell him that. This person is probably not your ideal partner.

ear Maddie,

Sometimes I think I'm just too nice for my own good. Hell, I know I am.

I went out this afternoon on what had to be about my two hundred seventy-ninth personal ad date. This one seemed a bit more promising than most: the guy wasn't bad-looking – that sort of tall, hollow-cheeked guy who looks like he needs a shave five minutes after he puts the razor away – and he'd been a player for a while and seemed to know which end was up. Hadn't spent any time around the organized scene, though, which always worries me a bit... but sometimes guys like that just aren't joiners, or they're worried

> *"he says 'i've been so lonely'... and i swear his eyes are glistening..."*

about getting outed, or something, so I pushed that concern aside and kept on chatting.

The guy – his name was James – obviously wasn't love-of-my-life material, unless they invent a way to graft on about thirty more IQ points. (Yes, I'm a size queen, but it's cerebrum size that gets to me.) But he was polite and attractive and friendly and masochistic, and, hell, Maddie, it's been a long time, and I know you know how *that* goes.

So when the waitress came to leave the check, I suggested that we get together again next week – which for most guys would be cause for throwing their hat up in the air and hollering whoopee, not that I'm all that great a catch, but there just aren't all that many single dominant women out there, you know? But this guy James just looks at me with these big, stricken pale-blue eyes like I'd just slapped him in the face, and says, "You mean we're not going to do anything *today*?"

Today? Jeeze, what does this guy think I am, a dominance vending machine? "No, I don't think so; I'd like to get to know you a little bit better..."

"Oh, come on, *please*," he says, and I swear his eyes are glistening a bit. "You don't know what it's like, it's been *such* a long time, and I've been so *lonely*, and you really do seem so nice..."

"No," I say firmly. "That's absolutely out of the question."

So, of course, ten minutes later, he's following me in his car back to my place – everything I've ever learned about negotiation and safecalls tossed away like a used Kleenex. Hell, I've just thrown away everything that Officer Kelly came to my kindergarten to teach us about not talking to strangers – all because a lantern-jawed masochist with big blue eyes pulled a convincing basset-hound impression over a mediocre cappuccino.

> **KINKY GIRL TIP**
>
> Clarify, clarify, clarify. If someone is asking you if you want to try an activity and you have no *idea* what they're talking about, ask them to explain it. Looking a little ignorant is way better than agreeing to an unknown!
>
> **KINKY GIRL TIP**

And even that's not good enough. When I have him stripped down and I start to tie him face-down to the bed, he stiffens. "I'm not into that," he informs me. "You have to hit my cock."

As you know, dear, I'm all about the backsides – what I know about cock & ball play you could fit into a condom, one of the "snugger fit" ones. But at this point, all I want to do is get this guy finished off and out of my bedroom – so I shrug and tie him face-up. He closes his eyes, which is absolutely fine with me at this point, and waits for me to begin. I slap his weenie tentatively and he lets out a little sigh. OK, I figure – just like a spanking, only on the other side, and maybe a bit more careful. I can do this.

Which is all well and good, until as I'm doggedly whacking away with a little strap and I notice that between his little grunts and moans he's saying something. I strain to listen: "I'm sorry, Pearl... Pearl, I'm so sorry... Please forgive me, Pearl."

Oh my god. This is the creepiest ever. This guy wheedles his way into my house, treats me like an unpaid pro-domme, doesn't even have the courtesy to *look* at me, then uses me as some sort of mechanism for purging some sort of weirdoid guilt toward some chick named Pearl that he did god-knows-what to (I really don't want to think too much about that). What the hell have I gotten myself into, and what do I have to do to get out of it?

The last question answered itself rather abruptly when, with a brisk stroke of the little strap and a moan of happiness, he squirted all over his hairy belly. Ewww. I grabbed a trick towel from the nightstand, wiped him hastily up, and threw the trick towel in the wastebasket – I'd rather spend $2.59 on a new one than use that one again.

I untied him as fast as I could and found something else to do while he put his clothes on. I don't think we said two sentences to each other before he left. I think he felt as creeped-out as I did. I hope so, anyway. In fact, I hope he felt even worse.

This lesson was one I'll never forget. I don't know why I feel like I came awfully close to something very bad happening, but I do. I kind of feel I got off really cheaply – a couple of bucks for a discarded trick towel, a couple more bucks on my hot water bill for the 45-minute shower I took afterwards. When I think of the stories I've heard of dominant women who've been attacked, I understand better now how such things could happen – and I think it'll be the proverbial cold day in Hades before a stranger gets tied to my bed again.

Off to take another shower,
Suki

The guidelines about safewords, safecalls, etc., are there for a reason. Yeah, sure, being wise doesn't always feel spontaneous and edgy and all that fun stuff, but it's a lot better than some of the alternatives. Go with your first instincts.

Suki didn't listen to herself, she let herself be talked into something she wasn't really into. (And she learned a hard fact that I've heard from a number of my dominant

KINKY GIRL TIP

Don't get your pussy waxed if you know you're going to be having crazy monkey sex that night. Sometimes it can get a little raw and even if you get off on pain, you'll be more susceptible to picking up an STD.

KINKY GIRL TIP

friends: a lot of submissive guys out there think dominant women are a special subset of pro-dommes who, miracle of miracles, work for free!)

Don't listen to those pleading eyes if your gut is telling you that you're not ready. Maybe a few more phone conversations would have brought out the fact that he wasn't really the sort of person that she wanted to be playing with. Maybe she would have found that there were some underlying issues that he was trying to work out through BDSM (something that can be done, but with great caution and preferably with a partner you already know very well). At the very least, she would have been able to set up a safety net.

As a general rule, it is not a good idea to play with someone the first time you meet them. It can be awfully tempting. You meet for coffee, the chemistry is there and you just want to rip each other's clothes off in front of the Starbuck's baristas. Try to contain yourself. Actually, if you hang out with the baristas, you will at least be in a public place. When you're arrested for indecent exposure or some such, you will also be reasonably safe. If you succumb to your lusts, or get persuaded by someone else's desires and take it private too quickly, then you may not be safe.

Yeah, people pick up strangers in bars all the time and take them home. Sometimes that works out just fine and sometimes it doesn't. The random vanilla pickup doesn't usually involve people getting put into bondage or situations where they cannot defend themselves. In Suki's case, she was the top and therefore not the one getting tied up, but she was alone in a sexual situation with someone she really didn't know who had an agenda she wasn't aware of. That could have ended pretty badly – as one friend of mine says, "Sooner or later, you have to untie 'em." And to make matters worse, Suki took her "friend" to her own place, which means he now knows where she lives. (She tells me she hasn't had any further problems with him, which is just plain dumb luck on her part.)

Get to know your partners, listen to your instincts, follow the basic safety guidelines with safecalls, etc., make sure you are a capable negotiator, make sure you're comfortable with what is going on. You'll still be taking risks but they will be conscious and mitigated.

The hell with Maddie – this is stuff *I* wish *I'd* known. I suck at saying no. I have hedged, backpedaled, weaseled out of situations, "forgotten" to return phone calls and done just about every other chickenshit dumbass maneuver available in order to avoid saying no. It isn't fair to me and it isn't fair to the people I am dealing with. I have not said no when I should have, and inevitably regretted it.

I have also been on the receiving end. People have just never called me back, not followed up, waffled around. That has always left me wondering what happened and feeling sort of up in

4: how to say no nicely

the air and frustrated.

People have also been honest with me. That may have hurt initially but eventually I was able to deal with it, work through my feelings, and eventually get some sort of closure. Personally, that is what I prefer. From them, I have gradually learned how to say no graciously and I end up feeling good about it, and the reaction from the people I am saying no to is usually pretty positive.

So how do you say no to people graciously? How do you maintain your integrity without hurting someone's feelings? How brutally honest should you be? Where's the Emily Post for perverts?

Just because we're transcending sexual boundaries doesn't mean we also get to transcend boundaries of being courteous and compassionate. There are ways of letting someone know you're not interested without being inherently hurtful. You may look at someone and think no... you're too fat, ugly, stupid, boring, egotistical, etc. The truth is that the chemistry is not there for *you*, they are not what *you* are looking for. Try that. *You* don't feel the connection that *you* want to feel.

This may seem obvious, but say "thank you." If you're flattered to be asked, tell them that too. If this isn't someone you feel that you want to develop a platonic relationship with, you can just leave it at that.

By the way, it's a really stupid beginner's mistake to come into the community and only look around for potential play partners, immediately turning your back on anyone who isn't the gender, orientation, age, physical appearance, whatever, you think you're looking for. The idea is to come in and meet *people* – friends, mentors, folks to hang out with. Get to know people and let them get to know you. Develop a network of friendly faces. The more people who know and like you, the likelier you are to get introduced around. This is the most fun, most interesting, and safest way to meet play partners in the long run.

So if this particular person is someone you don't want to play with but would really like to get to know better, go to the movies with, whatever, you can firmly say the chemistry just isn't there for you but thank you, you appreciate their interest, and you'd love to just hang out sometime. If, on the other hand, they're someone you simply don't like, a firmer "no, thanks, but thank you for the offer" is in order.

I asked a lot of experienced players how they said "no," and how they liked to be said "no" to. Here are some of the best answers I heard:

On saying "no" –

My rule-of-thumb for saying no is that the polite way to say no is to make it clear that the lack is not in the gift that they are offering, but in my own ability to appreciate/accept it. Hence, usually, some variant on: "Wow, thank you, that's really flattering. But I've learned in the past that it's really bad for me to do SM (and/or have sex) with people that I don't have a strong heart connection with, and at this point I just don't feel that connection with you; I'm sorry. I really appreciate your asking, though, and I hope you find someone else that it works out for you with."

Right before I became monogamous with my boyfriend, I had one date left with someone I had met through the personals. I was pretty sure this would be the last date I had with another person, and had a really great time with him. But by the end, I was sure I was ready to date my boyfriend exclusively. I turned man #2 down by telling him the truth: that he was re-

143

ally hot, but I was ready to become monogamous. And, as much as I think he was disappointed not to have another date, he was also obviously lit up by my compliment. And why not? - it was the truth.

My most polite no is, "I'm sorry, but I don't think I'm the person you're looking for." That works pretty well with personal ad responses and gets through to all but the densest people. The advantage of phrasing it that way is that it puts the "blame" on you, rather than the person doing the asking.

I don't think there's anything worse than saying "no" in a flirty style that is reminiscent of "yes" or "maybe." I've seen women decline invitations in this manner, then complain that the man won't gracefully take "no" for an answer. Argghhh!

A scenario that I witnessed not long ago was a new female submissive engaged in a conversation with a male dom she'd just met. The topic of conversation was her interest in the scene and desirable things she has, and has not, experienced. The interaction was lighthearted, while the dom explained how a scene might work incorporating some of her desires. She was in the conversation for the information, he was interpreting it as a negotiation. He did not ask if she'd like to play, he simply started to guide her out of her chair. She said, "I've enjoyed talking about this with you, but we haven't discussed pursuing this together. I'm not comfortable." She followed with a statement that she was enjoying the conversation and that was her need at the moment.

On being said "no" to:

The worst kind of response is no response at all. Did she get my email? Is she thinking about it? Should I send a follow-up email just to make sure she didn't delete the first one by mistake? A response almost as bad as no response at all is the long explanation about why she has to turn me down. Maybe she is being honest, but it comes across to me as contrived and dishonest. A polite response to the point are what I like. I can then cross her name off my list and move on to someone else who may be thrilled I am contacting her."

If you really do mean "not right now," then it's best to add "maybe later," or even to vaguely schedule a time, "could we talk about it next munch?"

I really really hate being equivocated to. "Perhaps another time," etc., just piss me off. If the attraction's not there, I'm a big tough girl and I can take it, tell me so – I mean, don't tell me I'm ugly or anything, but just tell me that you don't feel much physical chemistry with me; I can deal. I tore one guy a new one a couple of months back when he had responded with great enthusiasm to several rounds of personal ad correspondence until he received my photo, at which point he all of a sudden "had a very busy couple of months coming

145

up" — *I told him in no uncertain terms that he was both rude and a liar. (Yeah, I was PMSing; why?)*

Pretty much the best "no, thank you," I ever received was from a kinky poly woman who let me down so gently, it took me quite a bit of time to realize I'd been rejected. I told her I was interested in playing with her, and her response was something along the lines of: "Gosh, it's so exciting to get a play offer from you since I've always thought you were so hot and sexy. Unfortunately, I'm not looking for a new play partner at the moment, so I have to say no. But I think you're a totally hot babe and I'm extremely flattered." Now, it's questionable whether she was being completely truthful. I have always suspected that she thought a situation with me might take more emotional energy than she was willing to expend on anyone but her husband. And in the years since, she has never approached me for anything but friendship. But for days after our conversation, all I could remember was that she thought I was hot and sexy. It was one of the best rejections I've ever received and I always bear it in mind when I have to say no to somebody but I want to do it in a nice way. I left not with the sting of rejection, but with all these nice compliments that made me feel sexy.

*S*he looks back and think *I should have known.* With the frustrating clarity of 20/20 hindsight, she watches herself walk down the road of dysfunction. She wants to reach out to that girl and tap her on the shoulder, point out the signposts, the red flags fluttering in the breeze. Instead she can just watch her own lemming-like march towards the cliff.

She should have known with Ron. She still doesn't understand what was going on in her head. He started pushing at her boundaries right away. The first time he fucked her, he thrust inside her without a condom, even though she had told him her safe sex practices. He

she should have known...

stopped and was reasonably apologetic when she protested but that should have been enough. She shouldn't have seen him again. *She should have known.*

When he kept slapping her face as they fucked, "worthless bitch, useless cunt," even after she had told him that was a limit and really hurt her, she should have known. He would talk himself through his orgasm by telling her to go out and find him other women to fuck. She didn't like it... she frequently didn't like *him.* But she told herself she was just killing time, having some fun. Sure,

147

he was kind of a manipulative bastard but she was bright enough to stay on top of it and she had it under control. She occasionally had the troubling thought that she wasn't actually having much fun, that she missed her friends that he'd forbidden her to see, that when he wasn't around she felt sad and small, but she pushed it away quickly.

She should have known when he kept trying to re-negotiate boundaries when they were "in scene." He would wait until she got all soft and submissive and then he would push and push at the condom issue. "Don't you want to please me? Don't you want to make me happy?" She hadn't understoof the power of constant repetition. Despite thinking she had control of the situation, she didn't. She had lost control. *She should have known.*

He fucked her without a condom and it made him happy. In some dark secret place of her, she was pleased.

Then she went away for a few days and somehow, without his constant numbing presence, she regained her senses. It was like emerging from a fog. She went back, relatively clear-minded, and sat down to renegotiate her boundaries. They had to use condoms. He couldn't push at her limits when she was submissive. What was hap-pening was *not* all right with her and never had been. She was angry at the manipulation (angry at herself?) and determined to resist.

He was most distinctly displeased, cold and angry, distant, threatening abandonment. She should have walked out and almost did. The escape hatch was there, open and beckoning. But then he relented, agreed to honor her boundaries, turned all loving. *She should have known* but somehow she didn't. She believed him and she stayed.

She stayed with him for a few months which felt like a decade. She woke up one morning and looked in the mirror and didn't recognize the girl that looked back at her. The eyes staring at her weren't her own. She got the phone and went back to the mirror and dialed it with shaking hands. "It's me," she said, "It's over. I'm done."

"Wait," he said, "wait, I'll come over and talk. You're just confused. Let me..."

"No." she interrupted him quickly before he could weave a web of words around her, "No. I'm done. It's over. Don't call." She hung up the phone. It rang again and she turned it off quickly. She looked back at the mirror. The eyes looking back at her were filled with tears but they were her own.

♥

To the untrained eye, a lot of BDSM activities can look like abuse. People are getting tied up, beaten, tortured in all sorts of ways. It can seem like a fine line. The thing is, it's not. It's not a fine line at *all*. It's a whopper of a line... maybe even a four-lane freeway. The name of that freeway is CONSENT. People have consented to these activities, they have sought them out, negotiated them, and are fulfilling their desires. Sadly, most of my vanilla friends have been date raped at some point or other. I have heard of very few cases of that within the BDSM community.

Does that mean everyone involved in BDSM is a good person who plays by the rules? Nope. Of course not. There are bad people everywhere who do bad things. If you're lucky, you won't run into them. If you're smart and informed, you'll follow the safety procedures and listen to your instincts and avoid getting in trouble. Unfortunately, Maddie ran into a bad person, got carried away, let herself be pushed into uncharted territory, and didn't listen to her instincts which were screaming up a blue streak. She crossed over from what she had consented to, to what she was coerced into. This man knew some of her buttons, like wanting to please her partner, and instead of treating that like a valuable gift and a trust, he used it to fulfill his own agenda. Maddie thought she had the situation under control but she was most definitely wrong.

> **KINKY GIRL TIP**
>
> No, this one isn't fun – sorry, but I have to say it anyway. If you suspect you are being abused, get help. Your community will have local resources to help abuse victims. You can also call the National Domestic Violence Hotline at (800) 799-SAFE (799-7233).
>
> **KINKY GIRL TIP**

If something feels wrong, it probably is. If a situation is leaving you empty and miserable, pay attention to that. Don't just assume it's going to get better, he didn't mean it, he got carried away, he won't do it again, he'll listen to you *next* time. If someone is ignoring your limits which you have laid out clearly, you are no longer in the realm of "Safe, Sane and Consensual." Those are basic tenets, not just rough guidelines. When your inherent consent is taken away, through force or coercion, you are crossing that four-lane freeway and entering abuse. It is relatively unlikely that the abuser will suddenly take control of the situation and guide you back to safety. You need to take responsibility for yourself, no matter how difficult it is, and get some help and get out.

Some signposts to watch out for:

- Excessive alcohol or drug use impede the ability to play safely and also the ability to give informed consent.

- Being cut off or isolated from friends and family and the BDSM community. Isolation can be a powerful tool for an abuser. The lack of outside input can allow your perception to become seriously skewed.

- Strong expressions of jealousy or possessiveness. When Maddie expressed interest in playing with other people, she was punished.

- Verbal abuse or humiliation that is not negotiated or agreed upon. Some people enjoy it and use it in their play. Maddie tried again and again to stop him and he wouldn't. Being constantly told that you are "worthless" can start to make you believe it.

- A consistent pattern of discounting or ignoring limits. When SM or sexual activity is coerced

151

instead of negotiated, it no longer falls within the realm of consensual.

- The lack of a safeword. The bottom should always have the ultimate control of what is happening.

If you suspect you are in an abusive relationship, get outside help. Abusive situations do not get better, they deteriorate. The longer you wait, the more difficult it is to leave. Leave now.

Maddie is being vigorously fucked with a dildo in a dark club. All very hot and all that. Music pounds in the background, a pervert's theme song by Nine Inch Nails, "I want to fuck you like an animal..." She takes a deep breath and abandons herself to the song, abandons herself to him, abandons herself to the sensations curling through her body. She feels the ropes binding her down, the bench she is strapped to hard against her. His fingers catch her nipples and twist and she inhales the pain for him. She pulls against the ropes for the knowledge that she

he began to singletail her breasts by the light of a headtorch...

is completely caught, completely helpless, there is nowhere to go except where he wants to take her and she exists completely in this moment.

Suddenly it feels like a Mack truck has been rammed up her ass with no warning at all – not that a warning would have made the slightest amount of difference. It is a very large dildo, with very little lube, and it has been shoved in with great enthusiasm. Her whole body contracts around it, utterly shocked by the pain. She shrieks.

153

Now, normally, things being put there is a very hot experience... it's sooooo taboo and all that. Nothing quite like it to get the submissive juices flowing. This is just so *large*. She "yellows" desperately, trying to relax around it... if she just has a moment to adjust. "What's the matter?" he asks innocently... as if he didn't know.

"It... *hurts!*" she manages to choke out. Shock and sudden fumbling as the dildo is removed. As he unties her, she realizes he honestly *didn't* know. Quite simply, it was a dark club, there were a few holes, and he, quite by accident, got the wrong one.

He is utterly contrite and shocked, frantic with apologies. She collapses in giggles once the pain subsides and the realization of what had happened sets in. Basically brutal anal rape, by *accident*. Hard to get terribly upset by it: after all, he meant well. Shit happens.

... Another date, another man. Well... it *seemed* like a good idea at the time. Being tied to a tree in the woods and beaten. He thinks it is a brilliant idea. Maddie realizes what was happening and protests weakly. There are other people around... what if someone hears? In the fantasies, the bark was never quite so rough. She is also uncomfortably aware of insect life around her. In particular, it feels like something is crawling up the inside of her thigh. She shudders and tries to focus on what is going on. One really shouldn't complain in the middle of a fantasy scene... it just seems so impolite when someone is going to all this effort.

He began to singletail her breasts by the light of a

headtorch. She wiggles and… please let that not be a spider! The cracks of the whip seem to echo through the woods and she tries hard to stifle her moans. Suddenly the tip of the singletail catches the end of the barbell in her nipple piercing and pulls… she shrieks and he catches it immediately, doesn't yank it all the way back but only about halfway, tearing the sensitive flesh around the metal. Spiders are abruptly forgotten as a thin rivulet of blood makes its way down her chest.

"I could have put a band-aid over that piercing," he says sheepishly, trying to mop up the mess with a ragged Kleenex from a pocket in his toybag. "I just got so turned on…"

Days later, trying to scrub sap off her backside with nail polish remover, Maddie has cause to meditate on the stubborn gap between fantasy and reality, and the harsh unwillingness of Nature to negotiate.

155

... Another morning, yet another man. Maddie had been dating Nate for a couple of months. He really enjoys playing at one particular club and they have had a bunch of hot scenes there. They get along well. He's a hiker and they've been out hiking a bunch of times... wandering around in the fall foliage together. He's patient with her when she gets out of breath.

She wakes up from a half-formed erotic dream into a groggy awareness. Nate is on top of her, inside her. She pushes up into him, teetering between her dream and awareness. He thrusts like he's trying to climb inside of her and she meets his thrusts with her hips. She moans and he puts his hand over her mouth and she comes... mouth open under his palm. He shudders as she contracts around him. Suddenly he pulls out of her, just as her own orgasm is dying away, and she feels his come hitting her stomach as he holds himself above her. She sits up abruptly, horrified, and throws him off. "What are you doing?? You weren't wearing a *condom*?" She can't believe it. They've discussed safe sex protocols and he knows her limits all too well. He is still gasping for breath, "I just, I was so turned on... and you were there... and I thought just this once... if I pulled out... I wasn't really thinking..."

"You're right," she says. "You weren't."

She gets up abruptly and stalks to the shower, by now thoroughly awake and furious. She cleans herself off and pulls on her clothes. He is still stammering apologies as she slams the front door behind her and goes home.

He calls her the next day and she can barely speak to him, she is still so angry and feels so betrayed. "I *care* about you," he says. "No, you don't," she spits into the phone. "If you 'cared' about me you wouldn't have put my life at risk. We aren't fluid-bonded. If you 'cared' about me,
you would have let me make my own choices." She slams the phone down.

> **KINKY GIRL TIP**
> Bring Your Own Vibrator or BYOV. The best tops know the wonders of the Hitachi Magic Wand and come prepared. If you have your own old favorite, throw it and and an extension cord in the bag.
> **KINKY GIRL TIP**

One thing I freely admit is that I have made a lot of mistakes. A LOT. Not only that, but I continue to make them. Sometimes I repeat old familiar patterns. In my more creative moments I discover great new worlds of ways that I can fuck everything up. Overall, I am trying to learn from each mistake I make as opposed to shredding myself for it. I try to forgive myself and, if I am repeating a mistake, to catch it earlier on in the process.

In the BDSM world, we're playing dangerous games. As in life, mistakes are bound to happen.

Maddie's three episodes illustrate three different types of mistakes.

First is the well-intentioned fuck-up done in all innocence and with perfectly good intentions. This is basically the "shit happens" category. Sometimes you can negotiate until you're blue in the face, obey all the rules, and stuff still goes wrong. I've heard of earthquakes happening while people are playing. In Maddie's case, the guy just got the wrong hole. It sounds strange, but it could have happened to anyone.

This stuff can be hot, everyone's moaning and excited and oops. Everyone's fallible and we need to take some responsibility for our choices. Hopefully not too much damage is done, you signed the release waiver when you started to play with fire and hopefully your health insurance is paid up. Don't worry, hospital emergency rooms have seen it all.

The careless mistake is done when someone tries to do something they're not qualified to do, or forgets the basic rules of safety. They turn away to chat when they have a hapless victim mummified upside down. They don't really know how to tie those knots but hey, it'll probably be fine. They forget to cover vulnerable piercings. These mistakes frequently occur when someone is operating outside of their skill or comfort level. They can also happen when someone gets carried away. Be careful of careless people, be careful of tops who are showboating or playing for an audience. Speak up if something doesn't seem quite right. They might just not realize that the St. Andrews cross isn't nailed to the floor but you can feel it swaying. You need to be able to trust your partner, so pick trustworthy partners – and don't assume that your partner can read your mind; they can't.

There's a classic story of a careless mistake. It probably wasn't so funny at the time but it didn't happen to me and I think it's hilarious. A top tied his bottom to an overhead sprinkler in a hotel room. The sprinkler broke (duh) and activated the entire system, flooding the entire place and making everyone in the hotel distinctly damp.

The last kind of mistake isn't really a mistake. Well, it's *your* mistake for playing with the wrong person. The last sort of mistake is the willful disregard of someone's limits and well-being in pursuit of a fantasy of one's own. The sub has hollered yellow, and maybe red, but just a few more strokes will get the dom to the best orgasm

> **KINKY GIRL TIP**
>
> Don't wear your pretty bracelets and expensive watches when you know you're going to get cuffed. If you feel you have to, bring a Zip-loc baggie so they don't get lost in the toybag.
>
> **KINKY GIRL TIP**

of his life. The sub is bleeding and her hands are purple, but the dom is really in the rhythm and just isn't ready to stop. The sub has said she's not bisexual and that's a hard limit but the dom really wants to see her eat that chick out and thinks he can talk her into it if he pushes hard enough. The dom knows he's supposed to use a condom but is pretty sure he doesn't have any STDs and just wants to feel her all hot and wet around his cock *once*. See the section on abuse because all of these are warning signs that the person you are playing with is acting with malicious intent and doesn't have your well-being at heart.

Everyone makes mistakes. It happens. Some can be excused and worked out and some are inexcusable. You need to decide when to forgive and when to find another partner.

Is Maddie still making mistakes? Of course she is. She's still looking for the dom of her dreams, that man who will treat her like a princess and fuck her like a whore. He's proving to be somewhat elusive.

But her dreams are evolving. She has a much better idea of what she's looking for now and eventually he will turn up. She'll still have to kiss some frogs. But she's learning to be more honest with herself and with others. She's learning to ask for what she wants. She's learning to compromise without compromising herself. She's a little more discerning. Less and less often does

epilogue:
whither maddie?

she succumb to overwhelming lust at the cost of reason. She's learning to listen to her instincts.

That red carpet of possibility is still unrolling in front of her and she isn't stumbling on the wrinkles quite as often. She's learning that she is not the only one out there, she's not a freak, she's not going to hell. She's learning that her sexuality can be expressed in healthy ways, that there is nothing *wrong* with her. She had to stumble a few times to figure this out. She even had to fall flat on her face. You

> **KINKY GIRL TIP**
>
> Top or bottom, boy or girl, straight or bi, there's nothing that says you can't be a hard-core pervert *and* an incurable romantic! Hell, I want the thorns *and* the roses!
>
> **KINKY GIRL TIP**

may too. But she also learned how to laugh at herself – and that, Reader, is the gift I hope I can give to you, because as you and Suki and Maddie and I all stumble around in the wide world of kinky sex, we will all most assuredly need it.

First, check out my website at *www.lunagrey.com.* Then have a look at all these great resources:

Books

The Sexually Dominant Woman: A Workbook for Nervous Beginners by Lady Green, Greenery Press.

Screw the Roses, Send Me the Thorns by Philip Miller & Molly Devon, Mystic Rose Books

Some Women by Laura Antoniou (Editor), Masquerade Books

SM 101 by Jay Wiseman, Greenery Press

resource guide

The New Topping Book by Dossie Easton & Janet W. Hardy, Greenery Press

The New Bottoming Book by Dossie Easton & Janet W. Hardy, Greenery Press

The Loving Dominant by John Warren, Greenery Press

The Mistress Manual by Mistress Lorelei, Greenery Press

Different Loving by Gloria Brame, Job Jacobs, & Jon Brame; Villard Books

The Lesbian S/M Safety Manual by Pat Califia, Lace Publications

Sensuous Magic by Patrick Califia-Rice, Cleis Press

If the Buddha Dated: A Handbook for Finding Love on a Spiritual Path by Charlotte Sophia, Phd. Kasl, Charlotte Davis Kasl, Penguin USA

Organizations

(please see these organizations' "links" pages to find other regional groups):

Society of Janus, San Francisco *www.soj.org*

The Eulenspiegel Society, New York *www.tes.org*

Black Rose, Washington DC *www.br.org*

Boston Dungeon Society, Boston *www.bdsbbs.com*

Arizona Power Exchange, Phoenix *www.arizona-powerexchange.org*

For gay men: **Gay Male SM Activists**, New York *www.gmsma.org*

For lesbians: **Lesbian Sex Mafia,** *www.lesbian-sexmafia.org*

Other BDSM Resources:

Kink Aware Professionals *www.bannon.com/kap/* (a list to help you find BDSM-positive doctors, therapists, attorneys, etc., in your area)

San Francisco Sex Information *www.sfsi.org* (an all-purpose resource for answering your questions about sex and BDSM)

Caryl's BDSM Resources *www.drkdesyre.com* (great links for all kinds of BDSM resources)

National Coalition for Sexual Freedom *www.ncsfreedom.org* (a lobbying and advisory organization that helps BDSM organizations and individuals maintain our political and legal rights)

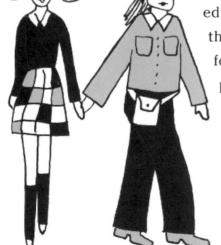

The Woodhull Foundation *www.woodhullfoundation.org* (an educational and advocacy group that advocates for the right to all forms of consensual sexual expression)

OTHER BOOKS FROM GREENERY PRESS

BDSM/KINK

The Compleat Spanker
Lady Green $12.95

Erotic Tickling
Michael Moran $13.95

Family Jewels: A Guide to Male Genital Play
and Torment
Hardy Haberman $12.95

Flogging
Joseph W. Bean $12.95

Intimate Invasions: The Ins and Outs of
Erotic Enema Play
M.R. Strict $13.95

Jay Wiseman's Erotic Bondage Handbook
Jay Wiseman $16.95

The Loving Dominant
John Warren $16.95

Miss Abernathy's Concise Slave Training
Manual
Christina Abernathy $12.95

The Mistress Manual
Mistress Lorelei $16.95

The Sexually Dominant Woman: A
Workbook for Nervous Beginners
Lady Green $11.95

SM 101: A Realistic Introduction
Jay Wiseman $24.95

Training With Miss Abernathy: A Workbook
for Erotic Slaves and Their Owners
Christina Abernathy $13.95

TOYBAG GUIDES: A Workshop In A Book
$9.95 each

Canes and Caning, by Janet Hardy
Clips and Clamps, by Jack Rinella
Hot Wax and Temperature Play, by Spectrum
Dungeon Emergencies & Supplies, by Jay
Wiseman

GENERAL SEXUALITY

Big Big Love: A Sourcebook on Sex for People of
Size and Those Who Love Them
Hanne Blank $15.95

The Bride Wore Black Leather... And He
Looked Fabulous!: An Etiquette Guide for
the Rest of Us
Andrew Campbell $11.95

The Ethical Slut: A Guide to Infinite Sexual
Possibilities
Dossie Easton & Catherine A. Liszt $16.95

A Hand in the Bush: The Fine Art of
Vaginal Fisting
Deborah Addington $13.95

Health Care Without Shame: A Handbook
for the Sexually Diverse and Their Caregivers
Charles Moser, Ph.D., M.D. $11.95

Look Into My Eyes: How to Use Hypnosis to
Bring Out the Best in Your Sex Life
Peter Masters $16.95

Phone Sex: Oral Thrills and Aural Skills
Miranda Austin $15.95

Photography for Perverts
Charles Gatewood $27.95

Sex Disasters... And How to Survive Them
Charles Moser, Ph.D., M.D. and Janet W.
Hardy $16.95

Tricks... To Please a Man
Tricks... To Please a Woman
both by Jay Wiseman $14.95 ea.

Turning Pro: A Guide to Sex Work for the
Ambitious and the Intrigued
Magdalene Meretrix $16.95

When Someone You Love Is Kinky
Dossie Easton & Catherine A. Liszt $15.95

FICTION

... But I Know What You Want: 25 Sex Tales
for the Different
James Williams $13.95

Love, Sal: letters from a boy in The City
Sal Iacopelli, ill. Phil Foglio $13.95

Murder At Roissy
John Warren $15.95

Haughty Spirit
The Warrior Within
The Warrior Enchained
all by Sharon Green $11.95 ea.

Please include $3 for first book and $1 for each additional book with your order to cover
shipping and handling costs, plus $10 for overseas orders. VISA/MC accepted. Order from
Greenery Press, 3403 Piedmont Ave. #301, Oakland, CA 94611 510/652-2596